PMR and GCA disease
A day journal of PMR and Temporal Arteritis
By Rose Lamatt
Copyright 2017 Rose Lamatt
ISBN:9781520486031

PMR and GCA disease
A day journal of PMR and Temporal Arteritis

Rose Lamatt

Also by Rose Lamatt

Just a Word
Is Life One Big Goodbye
Connected
Voiceless Cry
Carol: Rata, Rata, Rata

Beginning

When illness attacked my body in 2013, I had no idea what was happening to me. It came on slow, steady, then fast and debilitating. I felt death within my body and didn't know how to tell a physician or anyone else. They thought it was in my mind, fabricated. I began to wonder the same, but somehow knew I was sick, really sick. A kind of illness I'd never felt before. I thought at times I was going crazy and blind.

I felt my inner core melting, or I was giving up. Doctor said, it's probably depression, but I didn't think so. I had been depressed before and it didn't feel like this. I felt I was losing my mind. When I looked for the right word to say it didn't come. I knew the word in my mind but couldn't speak it.

Was it Alzheimer's? Dementia? What's the difference, they're both bad.

I found my legs didn't listen to my brain telling them what to do.

I felt something eating away at my insides.

I had faith, a Supreme Being, something higher than human being. But I started to doubt it with whatever illness I had.

It all started in 2013.

July 31, 2013

I spent two days in the hospital finding out at this ripe old age that it isn't *death* that I worry about. It's the fact that the medical profession needs help.

I found no one really listens, including some doctors. They make a decision and that's what they go on. They don't want to hear how you feel about their decision, or the fact they really didn't hear what you're trying to tell them.

Spending the first four hours in the Emergency room was an eye opener, even though it hasn't been my first through the years.

Three people were in my cubical/room, first me; then an older woman who had a glucose reading 600. When asked if she had diabetes she said, "No. My grandson has that." When her relatives came they said she *was* diabetic and has pain in her right side.

Next, the medics brought in an older man, maybe in his sixties, who I happened to see when they wheeled him in on a stretcher. Apparently he had fallen, "tearing up his leg" I heard him say, in a slurred voice. He had that dingy, unscrubbed look, long hair, disheveled, and dirty clothes. My thought, Homeless, since I had been around homeless in past years.

I lay on a stretcher listening to sounds around me.

A few hours passed and soon the disheveled man wanted to walk down the hall for a cup of coffee. He also wanted the television on. I smiled, knowing he was in a safe place now and would be given food, a bed and coffee. I often heard the nurse telling him to get back in bed, but he didn't listen. At some point the head nurse (front desk-watching nurse) ran out the door for something. At that, the man passed by my half-drawn curtain, and left without the limp.

The other bed became loud with laughter, and chatting. I listened, waiting for two blood pressure pills given me to kick in. Apparently the one I'd taken this morning didn't work, and the CTscan of head, checking for stroke came back negative. A good thing.

On the second day, doctors came to visit. I found some listened. Most didn't. I then realized how hard it must be for someone with dementia to try and tell doctors what they're feeling, where the pain is, or what they're hearing in their own mind.

I felt a little better on new blood pressure pills given me, and the fact I had made it through the night, after two hours sleep.

Lying in bed reading, I thought I heard someone calling "help". I wondered if my mind was playing tricks on me. But when I listened harder sitting up on the side of the bed, I heard it clear. Someone *was* yelling "help"....a woman's voice. "Help... Help...Help..." Not stopping, but on and on.

I wanted to walk down the hall and see if I could help the woman, but still felt lightheaded from new meds. I went to the doorway, hearing the woman in distress. My thoughts went to my dear friend Carol, one I cared for, who had Alzheimer's. My thoughts went to nursing home horrors she went through, and workers who didn't hear Carol, the day she fell and broke her hip. Or maybe heard her and did nothing.

In the hall workers were chatting above the woman's cry for help.

Am I the only one who hears her?

I spotted a worker in the hall sitting behind a computer, and said loudly, "Someone's calling for help."

The worker came to me, and said, "Yes, we know. She's at the nurse's desk being cared for."

"Does she have Dementia?"

The worker nodded. And I knew more work was needed for those with dementia, especially when they're caught in the medical maze.

It seemed to me if this woman yelling had a room with someone singing to her, or just calmly talking to her, soothing her in some way, instead of making believe she didn't exist, maybe she wouldn't be yelling "help" and be less agitated. I should have said this to the worker but I didn't.

I always thought I had the letter 'A' stamped across my forehead; because my mind is always open to Alzheimer's. Whether coming to me when I lived in a Homeless Shelter, or hearing them in condos I lived, no matter where I was. But I've come to believe this is a gift and feel bad when I can't help someone with Dementia or Alzheimer's.

I also found while in the hospital, you point to a face when asked a question, if you can't answer by mouth. "How are you feeling?" and you point to a face that shows best how you feel, the person points to sad or happy faces.

I'm home now resting, but felt the need to write what I saw and heard in the hospital. Probably because I live in Florida with many elderly, who will eventually develop some form of dementia as they age.

October 27, 2013

I haven't felt well for many months. I feel I have a fever. A hot flash comes and then I have inward chills up my back. Lately though heat flashes are in upper portion, waist up.

I feel hoarse as a chest cold coming on, but nothing happens.

Past two, three days pain in upper body, around rib cage, as if I've coughed a lot and strained muscles.

Eyesight seems blurry and eyes feel heavy or swollen.

Belly feels swollen with gas but nothing passes.

I wish someone would figure out what's wrong with me.

***

What is it like to have dementia? Just a word? No. Dementia isn't even a word. It shouldn't qualify as anything, especially a word. Words mean something this is a devastating word, a word that tears at your thinking, it can't be. I can't have this word. No, not me! That happens to others, not me. That happened to Carol, it can't happen to me also. What is the point to life if we get this word? Nothing matters anymore. Nothing. I'm not only losing my memory, but feel awful everyday: confusion, nervous, disoriented, not finding the right word for my sentence. So many other things besides losing one's memory. Why don't people write about this when they write about Alzheimer's or dementia? Why don't they tell you what it's *really* like?

***

It's not Dementia, it's a urinary infection better known as UTI. I've been put on antibiotics and after three days I feel better. I know what day it is. I don't feel confused or disoriented. Why didn't the first two doctors listen to me and find this? No, I had to go to a neurologist and find I had trouble finding the right words for my sentence. I couldn't draw the face of a clock. Oh, I got the circle, and 12, 3, 6, and 9. But couldn't figure what numbers went between.

I couldn't get my mind in order—the right order. It seemed jumbled, out of sync. I was sure I had a dementia of some kind. Little did I know there are many different types of Dementia. Shouldn't delirium fit in the Dementia category?

By the fourth day all feelings and bad thoughts were gone. I was *me* again. In my right mind.

Seven days on antibiotic's and I was able to walk in a store without feeling dizzy, with all those other symptoms.

But five days later, after last pill taken, I feel ill again. Fever coming on, hot, cold, the next two days, headache, day after disoriented, the day after that dizzy. All back, same feelings back.

Woke at 4a.m. this morning Feb. 3, 2014

Eyes won't focus. I look at the wall and my eyes go side to side, very fast. I switch and look at the window, still can't focus. I stay in bed, scared, closing my eyes. But even with eyes closed they don't feel right. Every few seconds I open them, still going side to side.

I take half a valium, hoping to relax. There's no way I can walk to the bathroom.

I lay still until 6:30am. By that time my eyes are better but yet not right. Not only that, I can't walk without bumping into walls. I'm dizzy. Very dizzy.

I call 911.

Paramedics come within minutes and I'm glad, someone can help me.

I'm transferred from bed to stretcher and taken to the Hospital Emergency Room.

Vitals are taken, blood pressure, pulse, temperature. Minutes later doctor comes in and I repeat again what happened this morning, eyes jumping side to side, and dizziness.

He checks my eyes, "Nystagmus" he says.

A new name. Never heard this one before, then says, "Vertigo," this one I know. "Usually caused by and inner ear problem," his answer.

He gives me a pill for vertigo, and within hours I'm allowed to go home.

By then I'm feeling no pain and just want sleep.

I feel hung over, like too much alcohol the night before. But I haven't drank since I can't remember when. Why? Because I hated the dizziness that went along with that vodka martini.

I lay down.

Two days later I'm at the ear doctor. "You have a virus that has attacked your sinus," he says, and puts me on Prednisone.

He walks with me down the hall to a special chair that swings me upside down and sideways to correct dizziness. I really can't tell if I feel better or worse. I do have a slight head ache so maybe it is a sinus problem. He does say, "You might want to check with a neurologist."

Home I sleep a lot on balance pills but when awake I feel jittery inside myself. I don't want to do anything, not even walk the store for enjoyment.

A week later an appointment with neurologist.

I'm shaking and glad doctor can see what's happening to my body, so I don't need to talk.

Doctor decides on blood work and nurse comes with needle, also says, "pee in cup."

It comes back UTI again. Puts me on antibiotic.

So, I've taken six days of Prednisone and now I'm on antibiotics for seven days.

I notice I'm feeling better toward the end of the dosage. Maybe someone found what's wrong again.

***

Where is my body headed?

Tell me again, what's the purpose of life?

Oh, right, You never did tell me what I was here for. Just an act of love between mother and father. I wonder if it would have been better if my mother had had a miscarriage or abortion?

It would have been better then living life as I've been living for the past years, neck fusion, heart attack, homeless, afraid to die.

For years I lived afraid to die. Now, I welcome it. But needless to say we don't get want we want, like dying without pain, or dizziness or eye Nystagmus. So I go on and on at this ripe old age of seventy-one, wondering what will happen next. Can my life get better? Can I get better for myself?

I write, thinking, this is what I want to be, a writer. I've written a few books, all having to do with me, my friend, husband, and children. But the last book I wrote was about me. Homeless, having nothing.

I think I feel better when I have nothing. Oh, but I need a computer to get the words out of me. Without a computer typing my words, getting the nastiness out of my body, on paper, on the screen, I would really feel bad.

I wish I knew where all this was headed. Where my life is headed. Where my body is headed.

***

Neurologist 3/10/14

Go over last tests taken, MRA's of brain and neck. Both came back normal, as normal as can be, being I was born with only one vertebral artery and a loop of some kind in the artery which comes out of the aorta, heart. The doctor says, "Nothing to worry about, people live with only one vertebral artery, and the arch in the artery coming from the aorta, normal for you. How do you feel?"

"Not good," I say. "Dizzy or spacey most mornings. Off balance. Also at times I feel I'm not sure what time of day it is and the space I'm sitting in. I know where I am, it's just that I have to look at a clock to see if it's morning or afternoon, being it's not dark outside. Also, times I'll be siting and all of a sudden a wave of depression comes over me. It comes hard and fast and sometimes stays all day or a brief moment. Very odd feeling. I was never a depressed person."

"How's your memory?"

"Not as good as it used to be. Names escape me, and I have to think hard what I want to say to find the right words. At times I can't find the right word and give up trying to convey my thoughts, even though I know my thoughts are inside my head. I just can't get them out of my mouth to someone else."

"What kind of health insurance do you have?"

"Medicare," I say.

"You should have a mental test done."

And all I say is, "What's it going to prove? I might have Mild Cognitive impairment? The outcome isn't going to help me."

Doctor still suggests mental test, which is about five hours long. I remember my dear friend Carol having it, while I sat waiting for her in the outer office.

Now, doctor orders more blood work, Cortisol, CK, C-reactive Protein, and ESR (inflammation) and an EEG of the brain. (new for me)

I say, "I have a feeling it's physical and not mental. Something in my blood. Something's making my brain not right, lightheaded, dizziness. I see dots at times, iridescent dots or lines, blue and green."

Something's not right. Period. I pray something shows in new blood work doctor ordered.

3/12/2014

Today I have results of blood work.

C-reactive protein high, CK okay, Cholesterol okay for me, but probably too high for cardiologist. We'll see when he sees the results. I'd rather not go on cholesterol meds again. Was on cholesterol meds for years before and after heart attack in 2011. They didn't stop heart attack from happening. I finally stopped them.

The ESR/SED rate (inflammation) is high, way out of range.

Neurologist suggests I see Rheumatologist, a new doctor.

All I know -- I'm tired of doctors. I'm tired of living if I can't write. My fun thing to do. I'm tired. Period.

I'd like to be outside walking, running, playing tennis, exercising, having fun watching, butterflies, birds, wild life, period. I wonder will I ever do that again, or will my EEG test next week tell them more about my brain.

I'd rather not go for the mental test that last four or five hours. I hope the high SED rate means I can take a pill for the cure.

Wish me luck.

March 28, 2014

Went to new doctor, Rheumatologist.

He asked lots of questions and only wanted answers to his question and nothing I had to say.

He pressed different parts of my body, asking, Does this hurt?" Mainly upper legs, upper arms, shoulders and pressed scalp, temple areas asking, "Any pain?"

I feel he gave me a good exam, then x-rayed knees, front and back, shoulders and hips.

I was there three hours, a lot of time spent waiting, noticing other patients. Most had walkers, lots of swollen faces, old and young.

"See me in a month," he said.

When I go back I'll find out results of tests.

***

April 5, 2014

Again I feel death. All around me. Inside me. I feel it growing within, taking my very breath.

I lay awake nights, wheezing, heaviness in my chest, hard to breathe in.

I wonder what it's like for someone with Asthma, or other Lung illness, that makes you feel you're being strangled. That's what I feel.

Doctor after doctor, almost every month, saying nothing and me telling my discomforts: dizziness, passing out feeling, swirling head, head pain down right side, heavy eyes, swollen eyes, eye lid twitching, belly blown up with fluid, weight gain, no appetite, muscle spasms in abdominal area, leg cramps/spasms, feet hurting, hips, shoulders and right groin hurting. Also constipation.

Every new doctor has heard this, and not one has said anything about disease, or what's wrong. "Maybe try thyroid medicine. Maybe try hormone medicine. Maybe try allergy medicine. Maybe try this or that." But no one has said, "This is what's wrong with you." Other than UTI or Sinus infection.

April 10, 2014

Rheumatologist's receptionist called, saying, "Doctor wants you to take Neurontin twice a day the first week then four times a day after. Also wants me to see Hematologist/Oncologist. Blood work shows high in certain things." Receptionist gives me new doctor's name, saying, "They will call you."

Again new doctor. Yippie. I hate this, and wish someone would come up with a name I know.

Not crazy about starting new drug. I already take five medications: stomach acid pill, blood pressure, Ventricle tachycardia, diagnosed back in 1989. And the wonderful thing, the side effects are dizziness and blurred vision. Aren't they two reasons I'm seeing doctors?

New drug makes me dizzier, if that's possible? I stop it.

April 21, 2014

Decided on seeing my old doctor, general practitioner, one I saw when first moving to Florida in 1985.

He's aged the same way I have, and gained weight like me, but not as much as me.

He spent time with me, but also called doctors I've been seeing, rheumatologist and oncologist, getting me earlier appointments.

I told GP what's going on and the doctors I've seen. He suggests I try 20mgs of Prednisone and see if anything changes.

All I said was, "Hallelujah, finally someone is listening."

"See me in ten days after blood work," he said and sent the nurse in to take blood.

So now we go forward again. Hopefully.

April 22, 2014

First day on Prednisone, two hours later I feel different. Right nostril cleared up and my chest could breathe. It feels light to breathe, not heavy and full of congestion, along with nasal drip.

I feel good.

I've gone to the store and I'm able to walk around without dizziness or feeling ill.

Next day, not good.

Hours after taking prednisone, bad head ache and dizzy. (same as before without drug)

April 25, 2014

Saw Hematologist/Oncologist. Scared about this one. All I see is word - Cancer. Cancer has gone through my family, mother, father, brother and my own child. Do I really want to know if I have cancer, now, at this age? It's debatable.

Apparently some blood work came back negative, to what it should be, something about too much protein in blood cell. I'm not swift when it comes to this kind of medicine. Some of the body workings I understand but not this.

The doctor turned out to be a she and I might say very nice. I found her easy to talk to. She sat next to me taking notes on paper instead of her eyes glued to a computer screen.

She first asked me what my problem was and as usual I couldn't think. No words came. I said, "I'll have to look at my notes to tell you." She didn't disagree.

I looked at my notes and read the same I've been reading to all doctors prior to her. Dizziness, headache across forehead into right upper side of head, hissing in right ear, pounding in head, mostly right side of head, numbness in back of head, and pain on top of head, aches and pain through muscles, spasms in muscles, sweats and chills, wheezing, hard to breathe at times, swollen eyes, nose and into head, and whatever else I had.

She listened.

I said, "Since my GP put me on Prednisone four days ago I notice a difference."

She said, "Medicine doesn't work that fast and it couldn't be."

"Well, I don't know, but I feel a difference, especially at night. Even though I'm waking every three hours."

We had a good meeting, and said she had to wait for the urine test to come back to tell her more. I go back to her in two weeks, along with other doctors.

The urine has been under examination for a week now, I wonder what they're looking for?

***

Now, a lot of this may be boring to the reader but what I've done is made notes each day how I felt, what I took, medicine wise, what ate. How the day went. It's up to you, the reader, if you want to read it. Looking back on it now in 2017 I found it very helpful. I hope you do also.

4/29/14

Eight days on prednisone

I think I feel better, but at times I don't. I'm still not good head wise, heady, sinus feels full, especially over the right eyebrow. Pain, headachy, right nostril burning inside, as in infection, sometimes all the way into the forehead and above. At times, very dizzy, but a different kind of dizziness, not vertigo. Loss of balance, or passing out feeling. At times can't stand at all.

My breathing is a lot better, chest wise. There is very little wheezing at night, and my air waves are clear and deep. Pain in body gone, which is great. No pain in shoulders, hips, knees, or anywhere. Getting out of a chair is much easier.

I notice I get hungry before a meal. I don't know when I last felt hungry. It's nice to feel hungry. Makes you feel alive, and want to eat.

I had lost my desire to eat.

Eyes are much better also. If I look into a light, or outside light, I don't see blue and green iridescent dots like before. My eyes seem to have better vision now.

Once in a while dull pain on right side head into ear and jaw, but I think that's even better.

I also notice a difference in urinating. It comes on real fast and strong. Not the dribbling that I was doing.

Also have a lot more energy. Not fatigued, as before prednisone.

Now if I could get rid of the dizziness and headachy feeling, sinus feeling. I'd be normal. Whatever that is.

Easier to turn over in bed. No pain or stiffness.

***

5/2/14

General Practitioner blood work ESR/SED reads 25. Dropped from 56. "Good news," doctor says.

"I have been feeling better," I say.

He says, "drop to 15 mgs. per day instead of 20mgs. And see Rheumatologist next week and see how he wants to move forward."

General Practitioner says, "I feel you have Polymyalgia Rheumatica and Giant Cell Arteritis. You will be on prednisone for at least two years or more."

I'm finally diagnosed. Finally a reason for the way I've been feeling for so long. Actual names for what I feel. In short, PMR and GCA.

I think I've had it for a long time, being I haven't had an appetite for many years along with muscle weakness.

My question. Did I get this illness living in the Homeless Shelter in 2009? Did it cause my heart attack in 2011? It's a thought.

Next day 5/3/14

Took 15 mgs of prednisone yesterday at 1pm. Didn't sleep well last night. Fell asleep around 9:30pm, woke at 1am, took ½ valium (muscle relaxer). Fell asleep then woke at 3am, and stayed awake till after 5am. Fell asleep and woke at 7:30am.

Took 15 mgs of prednisone at 8am, see if taking pill earlier helps me sleep tonight.

The only problem my symptoms are back especially head wise. No headache, jaw pain, and pounding on right side of head, ear noises (hissing especially)

But not feeling well mentally and feel panicky. I thought the prednisone was stopping the nervousness in the body. Now wonder if I stopped 20mgs too soon. Maybe I should have waited until the rheumatologist told me to. I see him on Thursday.

5/5/2014 Monday

Feeling bad this morning, took 15mgs of prednisone and still feel bad at 9:30a.m. Called General Practitioner's office and told receptionist, "I'm feeling bad after the decrease of prednisone."

She spoke with GP and said talk with Rheumatologist on Thursday about dosage and, "Yes" it was okay to take an extra 5mgs this morning to bring it back up to 20 for the day. I did, and then laid down.

Pain in jaw and right side of head, very nervous, eyes squinting due to light, even skin trailing sensations back last night.

Hope this helps till I see Rheumatologist Thursday.

Will take 20mgs tomorrow morning.

5/6/14

Took 20mgs of prednisone at 7am.

Not good all day head wise, nervous, sugar low this morning 75, so had half Ensure (vitamin drink) with milk, then blood pressure pills at breakfast.

The whole day feel jittery, then tired, sweats then chills. Body can't make up its mind how to feel. Laid in bed most of day, reading. I had more protein today versus other days. Almost two hours after I had ice cream my sugar was 154, hot face, head, neck, then sweats.

5/7/14

20mgs prednisone at 7a.m.

Again not good all day, until around 4pm. Then jaw pain left and head felt better. Not great, but better. I notice sweats after eating sweets. Sugar goes up, and down in the morning when I wake. 75, 85. After 2 hours eating 155.

Still constipated passing hard balls. Used suppository. Been like this for months and it concerns me.

Mentally not good today. Not thinking clearly, disoriented feeling, but not bad. Brain fog, I want to say.

5/8/2014 Thursday

Rheumatologist gave me drug for Thrush in mouth, 1 pill. "Take prednisone for another 7 days, then drop 1milligram every 7 days, until down to 15mgs. See how I tolerate this." Also said, "takes two to three years on prednisone for Polymyalgia rheumatic to leave body." See him again next month.

Feeling not good for 4 days then by Sunday I felt great. No headache problems except slight jaw ache. Still on 20mgs. Sleeping well. Only up two times a night. Have appetite, lots of energy, no pain, no aches, not heady, no headache. I'm getting Charley Horse in legs and gramps in toes. Maybe lacking potassium, I read on internet.

Monday again, feel great. Stood for hours in the kitchen cooking, without pain or dizziness. How nice.

Tuesday, woke nervous, heady feeling in morning. Still 20 mgs of prednisone.

Wednesday, not a good day. Heady, jaw pain, feels like sinus problems, like always.

Thursday, better today than the past few days. No jaw pain or heady feeling. 20mgs this morning. Raining all day, no burning in nostrils.

5/16/2014
7a.m. Friday, first day drop Prednisone to 19mgs. Three 5mgs pills and four 1mgs = 19. This for seven days then drop 1mg for another seven days, and so on, as Rheumatologist recommends.
Didn't sleep well last night. Woke 2a.m. with my old fast heart beat and high blood pressure. I have

not had this since being on prednisone for the month.

Took a while but fell asleep then woke at 6:30a.m. tired.

Head feels odd, I want to say congested but not sure. I did notice at some point in the middle of the night I was wheezing again.

3-4p.m. started to feel better, head and eyes not as swollen. Do have crunching in back of throat, like swallowing nuts.

5/17/2014
Saturday, heady this morning, nervous. By lunch time feeling was gone. Felt fine rest of day. Prednisone 19mgs today.

Sunday 5/18/2014
Woke feeling well rested. Last night, high blood pressure and not feeling well mentally.

This morning feel good, sweating a lot 7a.m. 19mgs of prednisone then 8a.m. breakfast, 9a.m. blood pressure pills. Noticed I started to feel nervous around 10:30am. Jaw, upper gums ache again as yesterday.

Belly very blown up. Still constipated for months.

Wednesday 5/21/2014
"Back on 20 mgs," Rheumy says. "Because symptoms are back."

Take four pills of 5mgs equal 20mgs per day.

Not a good day, nervous. Pain in jaw gone right away.

Thursday 5/22/2014
Didn't sleep at all last night. Fell asleep around 10pm. then woke at 2:30 a.m. and stayed awake until I got out of bed at 7a.m.Took 20 mgs of prednisone.

Friday 5/23/2014
Up 4a.m. sweating a lot. 7a.m 20 mgs prednisone.
Most of day, nervous and sweaty. Mentally very nervous, morning, then again later in day around 7p.m. b/p 141/84 pulse 62. Feeling a little vertigo. To bed at 8:30p.m.
Slept well up two times for bathroom.

5/24/2014 Saturday
Woke feeling bad. 7a.m. 20 prednisone, feeling very nervous, muscle tightness in upper arms and legs. 8a.m. b/p 168/87 pulse 78. Took b/p pills Diovan and ½ Toprol, same everyday then laid down.
b/p 9:30am down 140/84 had Ensure drink.
Don't like feeling so nervous and muscles aching and cramping even into toes.
11:30a.m. still high b/p 146/86
CO-Q10 200Mgs, supposed to be good for heart. Trying anything to be healthy, the way I used to be. Took pill with lunch: baked potato, broccoli,

chicken salad, peach. Even trying to eat healthier, yet thought I always did.

1p.m. Nervous and not good mentally, as if in a dream. Don't like this feeling. Upper arms still ache. Took ½ 5mgs of Valium, hoping to stop pain and nervousness.

2:30pm b/p 113/75 pulse 70, did the valium bring blood pressure down?

5/25/2014 Sunday

Slept okay last night. Woke at 3a.m. heart pounding in head, went to bathroom, high b/p, along with sweats. Took Diovan and Toprol (morning b/p pills) after an hour calmed down and slept, little.

Up at 7:30am took 19mgs of prednisone. Don't like blood pressure going up. Is prednisone causing high b/p? So you get rid of the pain in body and you have a stroke. Makes no sense to me, but then what the heck do I know.

5/28/2014 Wednesday

Rheumy visit. "Take Prednisone another seven days then decrease to 19 then 18," he says.

I just look at him.

5/29/2014 Thursday

Feeling okay today. Woke at 1a.m. took ½ valium back to sleep. Woke with tightness in shoulders and cramps in toes, settled down within the hour.

5/30/2014 Friday

Slept well last night, woke at 1:30a.m. took ¼ valium and back to sleep after maybe twenty minutes to half an hour. Slept till 7:30a.m. which was nice. Didn't wake with shakes or sweats. No Ensure in the middle of the night either. Took b/p pills at 7:30am, ate breakfast, then 9:30am prednisone 20mgs. Felt good all morning, relaxed, and thinking right in my mind.

Around 1p.m I started to feel heady, had some peanut butter crackers. By 2p.m. I was off the wall, heady, almost a headache but not, very nervous. I then ate lunch/dinner. By 3.p.m. I felt better.

4p.m. sweating.

6/4/14 Wednesday

Woke this morning 1a.m. not good. Very confused, disoriented, not thinking correctly and sweating. Drank half a bottle of Ensure and lay awake till 2:30a.m. Took ¼ valium and fell asleep. Woke again at 4:45a.m bathroom then fell asleep. Woke at 7a.m. and got up.

Today dropped 1mg to 19mg prednisone per Rheumy's instructions.

Not good this morning, spinning feeling, dizzy. B/P okay. All day dizzy. When swallow ears are cracking. Sinus?

6/5/14 Thursday

Second day on 19mgs of Prednisone. Felt great all day, no dizziness, no nothing. Felt great. I only hope this keeps up.

6/6/14 Friday

Third day on 19mgs of Prednisone, feel awful. Slept little last night, up every two hours. When out of bed this morning felt heady right away. Left nostril has blood when I blow nose, like this for weeks, yesterday not. B/P seems to be okay 120/70 so I don't know if it's prednisone or sinus problem. Wish 'they' could find out.

Headache later in day, worse 6-8p.m. going to bed.

6/9/14 Monday

Last two days have been okay. No symptoms of PMR/GCA other than sweats, dizzy at times, but not bad. I find a teaspoon of canned pumpkin is helping. Maybe the fiber in pumpkin is helping sugar spikes and lows? B/P been good, not too low and not high. Dreams are crazy, disturbing, but I forget them when I wake.

6/18/2014 Wednesday

Started on 18mgs of Prednisone this morning at 9:30am. this morning. I woke up bad, spasms in lower right leg and toes. Cramping has been going on for almost a week.

Also have developed black and blue marks on my arms for at least a week.

I slept well last night so it wasn't a case of not sleeping. I had slight headache later in forehead, along with nervousness, can't relax, lots of sweating or heat flashes. But cramping is bad. Later after walking in store I had bad cramps in toes, also yesterday. Feeling I don't have a brain at times, not thinking well. I've been trying to keep to a good diet: fruits, veggies, meat chicken or turkey, so I'm at a loss what's happening. Unless I just need to get used to lower dose or prednisone. Will have blood work next Monday then off to Rheumy.

Wide awake till midnight, then slept till 3:30a.m., then slept again till 7a.m.

6/19/14 Thursday

Woke feeling better than yesterday. Prednisone 18mg Around 11:30a.m. started feeling bad. Right side of face feels swollen, on into upper right side of head, slight ache in head, very nervous, jittery, shaky, unable to think right. GCA?

Ate lunch between 12 and 12:30 also took vitamin ½ 500 magnesium, potassium, calcium pill. Lunch-chicken, egg, greens, plum, cup of milk.

Felt better within the hour. Vitamins? Or low sugar and lunch helped?

Rheumy today. Start decreasing next week to 17 prednisone, then two weeks to 16. If I notice problems, especially in head, tenderness, headache, jaw ache, etc. then take extra 1 mgs and see if it stops. I can take extra 1mg pill after I've taken my daily dose in the morning. Like in afternoon if I find I have problems, headache, etc.

Next appointment in six weeks.

6/27/14 Friday
Slept well last night. This morning, slight headache, other than that okay for rest of day. Did take Magnesium around 3p.m.

Hissing in right ear tonight at 8p.m. and tired. Going to bed.

7/4/2014 Friday
17mgs of Prednisone today, first drop from 18. Felt half good most of the day. Not nervous, slight jaw pain but nothing I couldn't live with. Pounding in ear at night going to bed.

Slept well, up at 4a.m. then again at 7a.m.

7/5/2014 Saturday
Prednisone 17mgs, second day, not so great today. Pounding head this morning and in middle to night. Left side head pain. Different from the way it started on right side, slight ache. Jaw feels tight, after lunch 1p.m. sweats off and on, and still head pain (ache). Eyes feel slightly swollen. Wonder if the symptoms are coming back.

7/6/2014 Sunday
Took 18mgs of Prednisone this morning. Felt awful on 17, symptoms came back, especially in

head, and eyes. Felt better later in day today. And slept better.

7/7/2014 Monday
Again prednisone 18 mgs, like yesterday. Felt better again on 18, head not as bad as on 17mgs. Plus body doesn't ache as much, shoulders and hips.

7/8/2014 Tuesday
18mgs of prednisone at ten a.m. Eyes felt swollen upon waking up also very dry. Right hip pain still there.

7/10/2014
Slept well last night. Sweats started before lunch 12:30p.m. and stayed all day. 4p.m. got very tired and fell asleep for 30minutes.

7/11/2014
18mgs prednisone 9:45a.m. Not good today, little sleep last night. Fell asleep around 11p.m. then woke at 3a.m. stayed awake until time to get up 8a.m. Blood pressure up 140/90 took b/p pills.11a.m. still not feeling great.

Asleep by 10p.m. then woke at 2a.m. disoriented, confused to time and space. Took half an Ensure and felt better within twenty minutes, fell back to sleep, Sugar? Possibly? Woke at 7a.m.

7/12/2014 Saturday

Dropped to 17mgs of Prednisone at 10am this morning tried this for few days a week ago and had to up the dose because of symptoms coming back. Feel okay except twitching over left eye at 2:20p.m. Haven't been hot or cold.

Later in day symptoms coming back, headache over right eye. Just pushing on skin, spot aches all the way down to jaw. Symptoms coming back.

7/13/2014 Sunday

Prednisone 18mgs today, because of yesterday's symptoms returning. Not a good day today, nervous inside, blood pressure seems okay though.

Slept well, only up one time.

7/14/2014 Monday

Prednisone 18mgs again, feeling tired this morning after blood pressure pills. Lunch time magnesium pill, been taking this almost every day, helps with bowel movement. Went to store and walked fast and more than usual, felt good. Came home around 2p.m. and started cooking. Sweating a lot for two hours, and more. Drank coconut water. Blood pressure running around 120/80 pulse 65 to 70.

Bedtime blood pressure 140/87. Sleep at 10:30pm till 2a.m. then wake off and on.

7/15/2014 Tuesday

Woke at 5a.m. sweating and cold, slept off and on, out of bed 6:45a.m. blood pressure 120/82 took b/p meds at 8a.m.

Prednisone 18mgs at 10am, along with Ensure. Feeling out of it this morning, mentally. Thinking maybe UTI, even though no symptoms. Don't like feeling or thinking like this. Feel like I'm losing my mind, can't talk for myself. Making errors in words I want to say, said delete instead of dilate for eye. Will see eye doctor tomorrow to check on a sty and swollen lids, feel like full of fluid.

7/16/2014

GP doctor, but different doctor. The office has at least eight doctors. So I never see the same one all the time.

This one says, "Yes you have a UTI," and gives me script, Cipro 500 twice a day.

7/17/2014

Woke at 2a.m. and stayed awake for the rest of the night.

18mgs of prednisone, now on Cipro also. Belly very blown up today. Fluid?

7/18/2014 Friday

Woke at 3am took Cipro and stayed awake maybe an hour. Fell asleep, woke at 7a.m. Feel okay. B/P low 117/77 pulse 72.

Prednisone 18mgs at 10a.m.

Belly feels blown up again.

Around 4p.m. Not right thinking brain wise. Fell asleep on couch, woke worse mentally after dreaming. Checked sugar 122 within range of test, also woke heavy headed, eyes swollen.

6pm Hissing and ringing started in right ear, ate dinner, still at 8:30p.m. hissing in ear, better mentally, slight heavy headed.

7/19/2014 Saturday
Took Cipro at 3a.m. not good around 6a.m. pounding in right ear/head, had half Ensure. Better, sugar?

b/p 129/84 8:30 b/p pills
10a.m. prednisone 18mgs.

Feel like symptoms coming back, wonder if it's the antibiotic Cipro?

7/20/2014 Sunday
Slept well last night. Woke fine, sugar 77, feel fine mentally and physically.

B/p 119/77 waited to take pills
Prednisone 18mgs. 10a.m.

Around 11a.m not good mentally, nervous.

Later sweating a lot, but also working outside where it's hot.

Not great mentally.

7/23/2014 Wednesday
Blood work this morning and Urine test. Didn't take b/p pills till later, and felt fine. Wonder if it's the antihistamine I took last night. I got my old dizzy spell

yesterday when I turned my head. Quick dizziness, eyes also out of focus. Vertigo.

Prednisone 17mgs at 10:15a.m. down. See what happens.

4p.m. not bad today so far. Depressed or down more the word. I don't think that has anything to do with Prednisone drop, but who knows.

Slept okay, woke two times. Took antihistamine.

7/24/2014 Thursday

Woke okay. Slightly off, lightheaded after blood pressure pills.

Prednisone 17 at 10a.m. then out to store. Slightly lightheaded, weak feeling.

2p.m. feeling nervous, sweating slightly.

Slept well. Did take antihistamine.

7/26/2014 Saturday

Not great this morning, heady, lightheaded. b/p 121/76 waited till 9:30 to take b/p pills.

Prednisone 17 at 10:30a.m.

11:30a.m still not good, heady, nasal drip.

7/27/2014 Sunday

Slept well last night. Out to the store walking feeling okay. Sweating while cooking.

Prednisone 17

b/p is not as low today. No antihistamine last night.

Cramps in feet and toes today. Feeling nervous at night. Hissing in right ear.

7/28/2014 Monday

Woke at 5a.m. can't go back to sleep. Feeling sleepy this morning, but can't sleep.

Prednisone 17 at 10:15a.m.

8a.m. B/p low 115/72.

9a.m. took b/p meds after breakfast and drinking fluids.

Sleepy this morning, hissing in ear.

Antihistamine bedtime 10:30p.m, helps me sleep.

7/29/2014 Tuesday

Woke 5a.m. pounding heart beat through body, head, b/p 149/90. Took ½ Ensure and water, laid down, tried to relax. Finally 20 minutes later felt better, but wide awake, so I read, till time to get up.

8a.m.119/81 didn't take b/p pills, until 9:15 after breakfast.

Prednisone 17mg at 10:30a.m.

Not good today, head-wise, heady again, nasal drip later in day. Cramps/spasms in mid-section under left breast. (took Crestor cholesterol pill last night)

Seems like I'm wheezing every day on into evening and bedtime.

Later at night 8p.m sweats, heady, nervous, nasal drip all day, headache slightly, 8:20p.m going to bed.

No Crestor to night. No antihistamine. Did take ½ valium and protoinix for acid reflux.

7/30/2014 Wednesday

Crazy dream, woke at 3a.m. then back to sleep. Slept well until 6:30a.m.

B/P 124/92 higher than with antihistamine at night.

8:30a.m. now, after b/p meds and feeling okay. Nasal drip.

10:15a.m. Prednisone 17mgs.

Felt okay until 1:30p.m., started heady feeling, time to eat lunch. Cooked meat, potato, broccoli, ice cream for dessert. Better afterward.

Later in day, nasal congestion, sneezing, runny nose, wheezing, slight headache, hissing in right ear.

Dinner cereal and bottle of Ensure.

8:30p.m. Bed.

7/31/2014 Thursday

Didn't sleep all last night, wide awake. Took ½ valium at 3a.m. still no sleep. No congestion or wheezing, just couldn't sleep. Awake all day. Tired but couldn't sleep.

Prednisone 17mgs. 10a.m.

Rested all day.

In bed at 8p.m. reading.

8/1/2014 Friday

No sleep again last night, wide awake. Fell asleep around 5a.m for half-hour to forty-five minutes. Up at 7:30a.m

Prednisone 17mgs 10a.m.

Tired today but not bad, now 2p.m after lunch.

Wheezing today since morning.

8p.m sweaty, hissing in right ear, right cheek jaw ache, first today.

8:45p.m.Feeling nervous going to bed.

Fell asleep around 10p.m woke around 11p.m. totally out of it. Disoriented. Scared. Had some Ensure better within the hour, back to sleep. Pain in groin, right side like always. UTI again? Then awake, sleep, awake for the rest of the night until 7am.

8/2/2014 Saturday

8a.m. b/p 120/72 pills after breakfast.

9:30a.m Feeling lousy, hissing in ear, red face and red eyes, not good. b/p 144/87. Very bloated.

Prednisone 17mgs 10:15a.m.

Seeing General Practitioner at noon about blood work I had done few weeks ago.

Doctor says, Your cholesterol is high. I want you to take Lipitor 10mgs."

Not sure if I want to do this being one side effect is memory loss, confusion, which I already have at times, maybe from taking Crestor for years.

7pm. Dizzy, first today, right after eating dinner. b/p 124/77 pulse 70

Still have tightness in left side of neck and breast. Could be from reading at night, holding Kindle book.

Headache across forehead. Tired. Will go to bed early, 8:30p.m. b/p 109/72

8/3/2014 Sunday
Slept last night, not great, but slept.

Slight headache this morning and left side of neck feels tight, but not like yesterday.

Prednisone 18mg.10a.m. tried more this morning, because of the way I've been feeling.(bad) been on 17 for more than a week.

8a.m.b/p 119/79

Not good again today, but better than yesterday.

Was good until right before lunch and after. Heady, nasal drip, not good mentally.

3:45pm sip of antihistamine for nasal drip and forehead, see if gets rid of slight headache. Also thundering and raining out. Depression off Florida coast, barometric pressure maybe causing headache?

Not good later into night. Feeling out of it mentally, unable to think correctly, scared. Laid in bed reading until 11p.m, turned the light out and stayed awake trying to think in a right manor. Fell asleep around midnight then woke at 3am, lay awake off and on, mentally alright.

8/4/2014 Monday
Out of bed 7a.m. b/p 126/82

Okay mentally.

Prednisone 17mg at 10a.m.

Feeling great, went to store, tired from last nights little sleep.

2:30p.m. Not good mentally, foggy brain, storming outside.

Magnesium after lunch 2:30p.m. haven't taken it in a while. Just want to feel better. Can't stand this.

Hissing in right ear and left side of neck tight again.

8:30p.m. still hissing in right ear, eyes swollen, and tired. Hope I sleep tonight. Going to bed shortly.

asleep by 9:45p.m didn't wake till 3am. Haven't done this in weeks. Fell asleep again until 7am.

8/5/2014 Tuesday

Woke feeling rested, when up walking I felt good. 7:30a.m breakfast and b/p pills

By 9a.m, Not feeling well in head. Took b/p 145/89 high for this time of morning especially after taking blood pressure pills earlier.

Prednisone 17mg 9:30am.

Not good all morning, mentally, or physically, heady.

Bowel movement large, haven't done this in months.

2p.m lunch after lunch bowel movement again. Very different.

Magnesium pill after lunch.

Feeling better later in day and evening. Urinating a lot.

Bed at 9p.m. to read. Slept little, awake a lot.

8/6/2014 Wednesday
Awake a lot last night, bathroom a lot. Felt nervous inside body.
b/p 124/87 pills at 8:30
Prednisone 17mg 10a.m.
Feeling very nasal this morning, head fullness, ears, and nose, along with nasal drip.

8/7/2014 Thursday
Again very nasal in head, nose, ears, along with bad tasting nasal drip. Hissing in ear.
Didn't sleep well last night up three, four times.
Prednisone 17mg at 10am.
Slept little tonight.

8/8/2014 Friday
Awake early, b/p 135/87. Endocrinologist doctor's appointment, feel okay, got light headed in office. Apparently I have nodules on thyroid gland. Too small to do anything with. Too small.
Prednisone 16mg lower 1 mg today first time. See what happens. Felt okay, slight headache later in afternoon and evening. Storms around, barometric pressure?
9pm going to bed. Nasal drip all day and sneezing a lot at night 7pm. Hissing in right ear.
Slept very well woke two times

8/9/2014 Saturday

Woke at 7:15am well rested. b/p low all morning 106/71. Waited to take b/p pills. 10a.m 120/77 take b/p pills.

Nasal drip upon waking, still at 10:30 drip.

Slight lightheadedness.

Prednisone 16 at 10:30

Slight headache around 4p.m. thunder storms around, barometric pressure, or PMR?

Forehead headache later and mentally not good, depression almost.

7p.m sat outside instead of air conditioning, eyes blurry and still slight headache. Started sweating, went inside to air-condition.

8:30pm still up, watching TV, just not a great day.

Asleep at 10:30p.m Slept great. Woke at 5:15a.m. slept whole night, no bathroom.

8/10/14 Sunday

Woke feeling good, fully rested, not tired. Stayed in bed until 7am.

b/p 119/72 pulse 61 b/p pills.

Lightheaded, b/p low had egg with salt, and G2

Prednisone 16mg 3rd day on 16mg 10:30a.m.

Hissing in ear, had coffee hoping for it to leave but it didn't. Usually don't drink coffee.

Feeling okay, except for lightheadedness. Now 12pm

Out for lunch feel worse, heady, nervous, took 1mg prednisone at 4:40pm, headache, pain top of head.

Sip of antihistamine, bedtime. Slept well, 11pm to 5am.

8/11/2014 Monday
Slept well last night.
Prednisone 16mg 10:30a.m. Feel okay this morning. No nasal drip. Hurting a little right knee and neck.
Later in day legs, feet and ankles swollen.
Felt good until 5pm, then nervous and heady.
Bed at 9p.m. nervous. Read till 10:30 fell asleep woke at 3:15am. Stayed awake until 7a.m.

8/12/2014 Tuesday
Hardly any sleep last night. Feeling heady, throat congestion, nasal drip, eyes swollen. b/p 128/86 before b/p pills.
10am Prednisone 16mg
Feeling bad most of morning, very heady, eyes swollen. Laid down for a while when up feeling out of it mentally. Nervous, heady even aching in forehead. Even when swallowing feel ears clicking open and shut. Sinus?
3:30pm sip of antihistamine see if I feel better.
Sleep at 10:30pm, woke at 1:30a.m. and stayed awake. Took ½ valium, still didn't sleep.
Sweats, felt bad at 6am cramping, disoriented mentally off, Blood pressure way up, 155/99 pulse 80, took Ensure, coconut water, G2, feel a little better within half hour. But still not good.

Rheumy doctor said, "stay on 16, add 1mg if feeling bad. In ten days go down to 15. A lot of what I'm feeling is coming from prednisone." Then added if I get headaches take extra 1mg.

9pm bed to read. Slept good until 4:45am then awake for the day.

8/15/2014 Friday
Woke 4:45am.
Prednisone 16mg at 6am.
Fell asleep till 7 woke not feeling good. Still at 12noon not good. Head feels like sinus problem (as always) more this morning. Pounding in right ear and head, nasal right nostril sensitive, almost dizzy but not quite. Pain/ache above right eye brow into head, like before I started taking prednisone. Aching in right hip, and neck clicking (operation). I sometimes wonder if I got Giant Cell Arteritis from neck fusion operation? Cadaver bones and two blood transfusions. One bag of blood I got very bad skipped heart beats and the nurse pulled the needle out and stopped transfusion. I was so dizzy prior to neck-fusion operation I had no choice. But it seems I'm still dizzy two years later.

Finally took Prednisone 1mg at 3p.m. Also Vitamin D 5,000 units.

At five o'clock pain in head gone but feeling nervous, but all pain is gone.

6pm sleepy while eating dinner.

9pm bed to read. Slept an hour. Did not sleep all night and when I did I had crazy dreams.

8/16/2014 Saturday

Very tired, no sleep last night. Eyes feel swollen.

B/p pills at 8:15pm

Prednisone 17 at 9am. Upped the dose yesterday taking 1mg at 3pm. (maybe that's why I didn't sleep)

Got ESR/SED rate results today, reading 30, up from 18 six weeks ago. Been going up for two months. Was 10 at its lowest on 20prednisone.

Bad day. Headachy, nasal, sinus, slightly dizzy. Took Vitamin D 2,000 and Magnesium around 4:30 with dinner.

Slept well. Sometimes I don't think there is ryme or reason why I feel the way I do.

8/17/2014 Sunday

Slept well last night. b/p 116/82 pulse 60. b/p pills 8:30am. Feel okay this morning, before prednisone.

Prednisone 17mg. 9:30am. Upped because of 30 ESR/SED rate.

Sneezing and slight bloody nose this morning. Feeling pretty good though all morning. No headache.

3pm after lunch/dinner Vitamin D (2,000) and magnesium with calcium and potassium

3:15 starting to sweat for the first time today.

6:60pm almost done with dinner, started to get forehead headache, first time today. No reason why. b/p 140/81 pulse 79

By 8:30p.m. headache gone.

9pm bed, feeling nervous in bed reading.

Turned light out 10:30pm. Fell asleep, woke around 1am, then 3am, stayed awake till 6am, fell asleep ½ hour then up. Tossing turning night.

8/18/2014 Monday

Up around 7am, little sleep last night, toss and turned a lot.

b/p 116/81 pulse 71 8a.m.

b/p pills at 8:45a.m. with G2.

Tired this morning.

Laid down 10:30a.m. to 12 noon, slept little.

After lunch, 2pm not feeling good. Feel like slight headache coming on. (African dust blowing) but haven't been outside. Dry African dust comes to South Florida. Funny I don't remember this happening in past years. Only lately have I heard this term on the weather station.

3:30pm Vit D (2,000 and Magnesium.

Not good around 4pm, nervous, and heady.

7:30pm feeling tired from little sleep last night.

8/19/2014 Tuesday

Went to sleep early last night and slept well,10pm till 6:30am.

Prednisone 17mg at 10am.

Out to the store at 11a.m. Felt good walking in store.

Good all morning.

Slight forehead headache around 4pm. Could this be the African Dust coming from Africa? Been bad all summer.

Vitamin D at lunch time

Magnesium at 8:30pm.

Bed 9:30, Sleep around 11pm.

Woke at 2:30a.m stayed awake until 6am.

Bad night

8/20/2014 Wednesday

7am b/p 135/81 pulse 61, tired.

8am b/p pills

9:30am Prednisone 17mg tired walking around store.

3:30pm. Tired, tired, tired.

8pm bed.

Sleep 10pm. Woke 11:30pm Brain Dead, Scared, got up feeling like going to pass out. Finally settled down and fell back to sleep till 4am. Then again to 6:30, awake, not good muscle wise. Feel trembling, muscle weakness, and head not good.

8/21/2014 Thursday

Not good muscle wise this morning. Still thinking of last night when I woke brain dead. Scary.

8a.m. b/p 135/81 pulse 74

9:30am. Prednisone 16mg going down 1mg today,_see what happens. Wonder if last night's scare was prednisone?

2pm burning in right nostril (as in the beginning) also ache in head when I shake it or press right side temple.

Vitamin D (2,000) after lunch

3:30 sweats and peeing

4:30 ache in right temple when pressed.

Fell asleep half an hour, woke feeling tenderness above forehead and ache right temple.

8:30pm still tenderness and temple ache.

Going to bed, read or watch TV.

Slept well, up two times.

8/22/2014 Friday

Woke 7am feeling fine b/p 129/81 pulse 69

8:30a.m. b/p pills, still feel fine

9am feeling a little heady

9:30 feeling anxious, nervous.

9:45am Prednisone 16mg second day on 16.

Out for a while, not good head wise, feeling nervous, jittery, and thinking off.

9pm bed, b/p high 140/90, still off mentally. Sweats tonight, and woke 3 or 4 times.

8/23/2014 Saturday

Woke at 4am, stayed awake for a while, slept and woke at 7am.

b/p 121/88 pulse 69 b/p pills 8:30am

Very swollen belly, same as last night.

9:45am. Prednisone 16mg, third day drop.

2:30pm laid down and read, fell asleep till 4:45, deep sleep, dreaming. Woke eyes feel swollen and dark circles underneath.

8pm sweats sitting, slight headache center forehead.

9pm bed, reading, fell asleep around 10.

Slept until 2am, bathroom, back to sleep till 6am, back to sleep till 7am. Slept a lot today.

8/24/2014 Sunday

Up at 7:20am, head tenderness above forehead.

8am b/p 119/81 pulse 70

b/p pills 8:30a.m.

9:45 b/p 111/71 pulse 72

Prednisone 16mg 4th day on lower dose.

Feeling heady this morning, woke very congested, chest and head. Eye sight very blurry.

All day eye sight very blurry, and feel swollen. Headache at times, but didn't stay, thought it might be food, right before eating a meal.

Had a lot of fruit today. Steak for dinner along with vegetable.

Throat felt gritty all day.

2:30pm Vitamin D (2,000)

8pm, tired, tired most of day, B/P has been low all day, 110/80. Had salt for dinner with steak.

Very little sweating, maybe three times.

Lower back hurts/aches, and very blown up belly.

8:30pm. Bed

Didn't sleep well, slightly dizzy getting up to bathroom, then wheezing, difficulty breathing all night. Felt belly up into chest.

8/25/2014 Monday
Tired this morning, slept little due to breathing difficulty, wheezing most of the night, and feeling dizzy, b/p 98/54, (very low)
Morning 8:30am b/p 124/76 b/p meds. Tired, up very early.
10am Prednisone 16mg 5th day.
Bacon, egg and decaf coffee.
11am feeling better than earlier, no wheezing and headiness gone, no congestion. Why? Bacon? Salt? Protein egg?
1pm still feel okay.
2pm lunch, chicken, bean salad, fruit.
3pm feeling sandpaper on tongue back down into throat (vinegar on bean salad? Green tea? Ice cream? Stomach Gerd? Which is causing wheezing also? Haven't had wheezing since out of bed this morning.
Bed 9pm.
Woke at 4am stayed awake, fell asleep around 5am again till 6:30.

8/26/2014 Tuesday
Didn't sleep well last night, sweats and up.
7:30am b/p 133/91 pulse 69
8am b/p pills
Tired this morning, eyes feel swollen slightly.

9:45am Prednisone 16mg sixth day.

Not good, tired most of day, eyes feel swollen, slightly dizzy, off balance, belly blown up all day.

8:30pm, sweats

Going to bed, tired.

Asleep by 9:30pm, woke 2 times then up at 6am.

8/27/2014 Wednesday

Woke, rested, belly still large, wheezing.

8am b/p 125/78

8:30 b/p pills

Neck hurts left side back. Nasal drip this morning.

9:45am Prednisone 16mg seventh day.

11:30 slight forehead headache, nasal.

1pm. Bloody nostril (left side), get this a lot.

4:45pm still have forehead headache (hurts when I press it) also left nostril bleeding.

Not good, dizzy also.

Laid down a while and fell asleep. When I woke headache gone, and bleeding nose stopped.

9pm tired, going to bed. (no headache, wheezing, bloody nose). Slept from 11pm till 6am, up one time.

8/28/2014 Thursday

Pain in thighs, last night and yesterday. Woke around 6am, wheezing. Muscles feel jittery, took some Ensure and water, laid back down, felt better up at 7am

b/p 121/81

b/p pills 8:30

10am Prednisone 16mg.

Eyes blurry, swollen, left side of neck hurting.

12:30pm Finished lunch chicken, pineapple, cheese, melt. 2pm, ice cream.

4pm laid down not feeling good mentally, confusion, disoriented, fell asleep for an hour. Woke, confused.

Possible low sugar attack before and after nap, had ice cream at 2pm.

Dinner 6:30pm, chicken, potato's, salad, apple pie and ice cream.

8:30pm bad, very nervous, b/p up, but mostly mentally not good, more disoriented feeling, peeing more, or feeling to pee often, UTI infection back?

Going to bed shortly, not feeling good mentally. I will read.

Fell asleep around 11pm, woke at 3:30am stayed awake off and on till 6am.

8/29/2014 Friday

Woke this morning feel okay, but tired. Eyes swollen, b/p 119/81 pulse 69 (took b/p pills at 9am a little late)

Yesterday's mental thinking could have been from cheese I had on sandwich for lunch. At times cheese brings on headaches.

10:15am Prednisone 16mg

Did a lot of work with eyes, reading, 5pm feeling like Nystagmus slightly, took glasses off and laid down. Fell asleep for fifteen minutes and felt better.

Slight headache after eating dinner 7pm possible walnuts.

8:45pm bed to read. Lights off 10:30pm after reading.

Bad night, woke at 1:30am bathroom, back to sleep, woke again feeling well rested at 3:30am, didn't go back to sleep, wide awake, but stayed in bed. Slept maybe half an hour up at 7am.

8/30/2014 Saturday

Tired this morning, bad night last night. b/p 119/81 pulse 69. Took blood pressure pills around 8:30a.m. then Prednisone 16mg at 10a.m. Did nothing all morning, feeling very tired.

Around 4p.m hissing in right ear started and eyes feel swollen.

7:30pm after dinner and heart pills I didn't feel mentally right. Couldn't figure the time of day. Feels like it should be earlier. I'm disoriented, confused, and scared, hot and sweaty.

8:45pm. top of head feels very hot and hissing ear. Can't stand this feeling. I'm going to bed to read, get my mind on something besides what my body is doing.

10pm stopped reading and took Protonix for acid reflux. Been taking it for a years. After fell asleep. Woke around 1a.m., then again 3:30a.m.

8/31/2014 Sunday

Woke at 6:15am feeling funny. Ache outside of both ankles into the bone. Laid in bed for a while then up to bathroom, feel jittery, shaky, and then started to feel as I have before, like having a stroke, left arm feels odd, left leg, and outside toes on left foot feel numb, and face red. Checked b/p 155/89 pulse 79

Drank coconut water and regular water, some Ensure. After fifteen minutes b/p down 133/81 pulse 74. Ate breakfast, cereal, banana with milk, drank more water. Took b/p pills. b/p down 121/80

10:30am Prednisone 16mg with egg and sunflower seed butter and bread. Feeling better.

Eyes blurry today.

Sleepy later in day, but didn't sleep.

Dinner late, oatmeal.

8pm, still sleepy, could go to bed and sleep, but will wait until 9, because I just got done finishing dinner.

Slept off and on tonight, 11 to 6am. No sweating, or nervousness, just awake, then after six I fell asleep for an hour.

9/1/2014 Monday

Woke with aches around ankles again, spasms in feet. b/p 119/81 pulse 72.

Lightheaded this morning, and hissing in right ear. Also ache when press right temple. I noticed this the other day, in the morning.

10am Prednisone 16mg with something to eat.

Not good this morning. Headache middle of forehead, left cheek feels swollen and not good mentally. 112/72 b/p eleven o'clock morning.

After lunch 1pm headache worse and hissing in ear.

Also burning in right nostril.

7:30pm not a good day, headache, hissing in ear, jaw pain and sinus type headache. Bad all around.

Going to bed early 8:30pm

Read until 11pm.

Woke at 3am, while walking to bathroom dizzy, back to bed dizzy. Feels like bed is moving. Stayed awake till morning. Chirping in right ear and hissing.

9/2/2014

b/p high 168/97 at 6am. Took morning b/p pills Diovan and Metoprolol ½ pill.

10am b/p 117/72 still dizzy, but not as bad as early morning and last night.

10am prednisone 16

Face feels like having a stroke. One side feels numb not working together with other side of face.

2pm after lunch, still not good, slight dizziness, hissing in ear, pounding also. Nasal drip, terrible taste in mouth and blood from left nostril.

b/p 113/74 pulse 72

Fell asleep around 4p.m. for half hour, felt little better when up, not dizzy.

Slight headache after eating dinner at 6:30pm. Still nasal drip, hissing in right ear, b/p 124/81 slightly dizzy.

8pm sweats, had little sweats today, had many after waking at 3a.m. this morning.

Going to bed early tonight, 8:30pm

Slept well up 3 times, but back to sleep after.

9/3/2014 Wednesday

Woke 5:45a.m. feeling okay. Woke cold then sweats.

b/p 134/82 took pills after eating.

Up all morning, out of the house, feel okay, not dizzy, no headache, eyes even feel able to look at sunlight, without seeing lines or blind spots. Nasal drip, but not bad, or distasteful.

10:15a.m. Prednisone 15mg first day.

12:30 slight headache, also dizzy surges, time for lunch.

Not a good afternoon. 2:30 afternoon laid down and fell asleep right away, woke with a start 3pm, words in line going across fast in my eyesight.

Now up with slight headache. Not much to eat today.

Dinner 6pm slight headache. After eating headache gone. Feeling okay at 8pm

Bed early again tonight, 8:30pm

Sleep by 11pm awake at 2:30a.m. took ½ valium fell back to sleep until 4 then stayed awake.

9/4/2014 Thursday

Out of bed at 6a.m. awake since 4a.m.

b/p 122/78 pills with breakfast 6:45am.

Very tired, not good this morning, feeling like stroke again. Right cheek and right foot, leg feeling numb. All morning, better when standing up, sitting my feet are going numb.

My old General Practitioner today at 10am. Blood pressure in office 160/88.

Very nervous in office and not good mentally, can't think correctly. He took blood work SED rate along with other testing. He suggested I see the Neurologist. He said it might be Multiple Sclerosis, and mentioned a spinal tap.

I asked, if he thought this could be caused by taking Prednisone? He didn't think so.

11:15am. Prednisone 15mg, second day on 15, late today

1pm, still not great home, hissing in right ear, getting ready to eat lunch. Had Ensure, peanut butter crackers.

Lunch around 1:30pm

Slept fifteen minutes between 3 and 4p.m. woke slightly confused and scared.

5:30pm sweats, first time today, been cold all day.

127/94 pulse 70

7pm sweats and panic come on for no reason.

Moved bowels 3 times today, loose the last time, also stomach cramps, and muscle spasms.

Going to bed early tonight. Eyes have not been swollen all day. They usually are. I wonder is it the drop in prednisone?

Been scared, and depressed a lot today. Feel I'm losing hope.

When diagnosed with PMR/GCA I figured this is why I felt so bad and then prednisone is making me feel worse. But General Practitioner said, he didn't think so, not the numbness in cheek, face and toes.

Slept little tonight. Worried I might have Multiple Sclerosis as doctor said.

9/5/2014 Friday

Woke around 4:30am, tired, fell back to sleep. Woke again around 6am to bathroom. When up I felt woozy, falling almost. Went to bathroom, feeling heart beating hard, face very red.

Blood pressure, 187/101 pulse 98 (too high). Took b/p pills, Diovan and Toprol ate some cereal and drank water.

Feeling very shaky.

Went to ER Hospital. Couldn't stop shaking.

In Emergency Room b/p 200/101. Questions asked, "why am I shaking?" I didn't have answer, been doing it for months, not all the time, but at times. They gave me Ativan (relaxant) and Metoprolol (generic for Toprol). I got dizzy or woozy, eyes almost crossing, and stopped shaking. Very relaxed. b/p down, 150'/80's then when home three hours later 11:30am b/p 119/74.

Now 2:15pm still feeling relaxed, not crazy like I've been and shaking. Brain even feels better thinking. Not depressed, confused, or disoriented to time and space.

5pm b/p 129/84 eating dinner. Shaky a little, took b/p pills early.

8pm, tired, going to bed. Feel okay.

Slept through until 4am, then back to sleep till 7am.

9/6/2014 Saturday

Woke feeling okay. Bathroom, urine slightly orange color instead of green/yellow.

8am. b/p 135/82 pills with breakfast.

8:30 feel pounding on right side ear. Also very congested, nasal drip and throat congested.

Wheezing.

9:30am prednisone 15mg

106/72 b/p

2:30 feeling heady, hissing in right ear.

4-5p.m. laid down, slept few minutes.

5:30 b/p 157/84 pulse 79

Jittery, jumpy, nervous inwardly, hissing in right ear.

6pm Dinner b/p pills verapamil, Plavix, aspirin 81mg

Tired of feeling this way.

8pm b/p 123/79 pulse 70 still hissing in right ear, not jittery.

Going to bed shortly.

9pm b/p 158/87 pulse 71 feeling not right. Drank some coconut water. Why? For potassium, 'they' say we need it.

In bed I read and fell asleep, woke 4 times in the night.

9/7/2014 Sunday

Woke 5:30am, bathroom, feel shaky. Back to bed.

Up at 7:15, off balance, not real shaky.

b/p 120/81 pulse 72, breakfast, b/p pills

9:45 Prednisone 15mg

11:30am not great mentally, wobbly, off balance, all morning. b/p okay.

Went to store 12:45pm felt okay, feet bothering me a little, numbness on outside of right foot.

Been a good day.

8pm. 124/78 pulse 72

Felt pretty good all day, except for this morning.

Going to bed, tired, relaxed really, and read a book.

9/8/2014 Monday

Fell asleep early last night 9pm, woke at 12:30am feeling like I'm having a stroke. Left and right side of face felt not together (hard to explain) laying on right side when I woke. Pounding in right ear. Lay awake for a while, drank water and some Ensure. Fell back to sleep. Woke around 4am, okay.

Up at 7am. Left arm, midway, feels numb.

B/P 128/79 pulse 79

8am b/p pills Diovan (not generic I've been taking for weeks).

10am Prednisone 15mg.

Not good this morning, feeling like last night, stroke feeling. Also can't think correctly.

11am b/p 145/88

Lunch at 1pm, feeling hungry.

2pm not good again, nervous, heady, hissing in ear.

b/p 126/72 pulse 79

Cold this afternoon, laid down 5-6pm

6:15pm dinner

6:30 b/p pills and Plavix, verapamil, aspirin.

7:15pm dizzy surge while sitting. Then standing doing dishes slightly off and head pain, hissing. Sweats.

Had nuts today. (possible migraine)

Bed 8:45pm to read. Asleep by 11pm woke around 2am, stayed awake all night.

9/9/2014 Tuesday

No sleep since 2am. Pounding in right ear, sweating, and not good mentally, thinking crazy, uneven, can't explain.

8am b/p 113/80 pulse 69

Mid-section muscle cramps under left breast while stretching.

8:30 b/p pills (Diovan and Metoporolol)

10am Prednisone 15mg. 7days on fifteen

2pm Cramping in med-section under breast.

Right foot cramping, left outside foot/ankle and aches.

Neurologist at 4pm, b/p 170/90.

She wants me on 10mgs of prednisone.

She thinks numbness I'm getting is from the neck, (hurting on left side past few days) Also gave me Ativan (lorazapam) 0.5 for nerves and sleep.

She said maybe if I were sleeping better my head and brain would feel better. Didn't take Ativan. Don't like the side effects. They're worse than what I'm experiencing already.

7:30pm b/p 119/80 pulse 79

Bed by 9pm sleep by 10, woke at 12am, fell back to sleep, woke at 4am, cramping (stiff) right arm, aching.

9/10/2014 Wednesday

Woke right arm aching. Otherwise okay.

8:15am b/p 116/80 pulse 70

b/p pills 8:45am

10am heady, lightheaded. b/p 106/76 pulse 79

10am Prednisone 15mg, 8th day.

Had peanut butter crackers, yogurt and water, still heady, (low b/p) headachy also, but okay mentally.

12pm lunch, then out to store, feel lousy, headache across forehead (eye brows), burning in right nostril, lightheaded, slight dizziness.

Found out blood work from General Practitioner's office ESR from Sept. 4th reads 50, higher than 30 last month.

5pm still not great, forehead headache, hissing in ear.

Not good tonight, same as all day. Top right above eye brow pain, eyesight very blurry. (GCA?)

Bad day

9pm going to bed.

Slept from 9:30pm to 12:30am then wide awake rest of the night.

9/11/2014 Thursday

Very little sleep last night. Tired. Left side of neck hurts.

8am b/p 123/88 pulse 70

b/p pills with breakfast

Rheumatologist today says up Prednisone to 20mg for ten days, then back down to 15mgs.

So I'm back what I started at, 20mgs. Is this drug helping me at all?

11:45am Prednisone 20mgs first day again.

1pm, not good feeling woozy (maybe due to no sleep) feeling heady, and right side upper head aching. Even pressing right side of forehead there's pain.

Laid down, but can't sleep.

2:45pm ½ Ativan to sleep, relax. Feel nervous and eyesight not good, very blurred, even blind spots in right eye, while reading.

4pm up, couldn't sleep, but feel a little better, not as nervous. Pain across mid-section, like this morning lying in bed, when up moving around.

Muscle pull from moving on Rheumatologist's table during bone scan, maybe?

6pm took b/p pills verapamil, Plavix, aspirin early.

Sweats after eating dinner.

9pm bed. Read till 9:30, took Protonix (stomach acid) like every night.

Slept till 12 midnight then awake. Took other half of Ativan and fell asleep till 5am. Slept well.

9/12/2014 Friday
Slept well last night.
b/p 120/81 pulse 72 feeling relaxed.
Head still aches on right upper side.
b/p pills with breakfast, Valsartan and Toprol ½ .

Cramps in stomach most of the morning, and bathroom lots of peas, then light color peas, maybe corn from last night's dinner.

10am, Prednisone 20mg second day.

1:30pm after lunch feel nervous, jumpy, belly blown up, pounding in right ear.

2:45pm. ½ Ativan for nervousness.

Slept from 4-5pm, woke slightly out of it, mentally.

8pm tired, slight hissing in right ear. 119/78 pulse 79.

9pm. bed to read.

Slept from 10pm to 1am, took Ativan, fell back to sleep and woke at 4am.

9/13/2014 Saturday

Up standing at 6:30am, nervous, shaky.
b/p 128/82 pulse 70
breakfast then Diovan and Toprol
8am still slightly nervous, but not shaky.
9:30a.m Prednisone 20mg third day
Not great this morning, laid down 10-11am. fell asleep.
Cramps in toes and feet getting up from bed.
1pm lunch, magnesium/calcium/potassium vitamin.
4pm vitamin D, 2,000 with milk, potato chips, pretzels. Having salt to see if there's a difference. I read where salt brings on flares for MS patients. Do I have MS and they've diagnosed me wrong with PMR and GCA?
Sweats in afternoon.
5:30pm. pounding in right side of head.
Dinner, chicken, broccoli.
Bed at 8:30pm. to read.
Slept from 10:30pm. to 12am. woke hard to breath, took ½ Ativan, fell off to sleep.

It's either sleep with Ativan, feel hung over, drag myself around most of the day, or don't take Ativan and be nervous and jittery on Prednisone. I think I'm learning the process.

Sunday 9/14/2014
Woke 7am. up, ate breakfast 7:30am. b/p 121/83 pulse 72
b/p pills at 8:15am.

Tired.

Prednisone 20mg at 9:30am. fourth day

Went to bed, read a while then tried sleeping, trouble breathing again, like last night. Belly bloated.

1:30pm. magnesium/potassium/calcium vitamin.

Not good today, hard to breathe, fast heart rate high 80's, high for me.

b/p 114/72 pulse 62

Not good mentally, hung over feeling. I guess from Ativan last night.

Felt better around 4:30pm., mentally.

7:30pm after dinner at 6:30. Feeling better, but tired, not passing gas, no normal bowel movements again except small balls, with white specks in stool.

Went to bed around 9pm. Read till 10:30pm., took ½ valium and slept till 2:30am., then fell back to sleep and slept till 5:45am.

9/15/2014 Monday

Woke early 5:45am., feeling well. No problems in the middle of the night with ½ valium. I think I like Valium better than Ativan. Am I a junky? Stuck on drugs?

When awake I have cramping in feet, slight. Drank water and some Ensure.

8am b/p 126/87 pulse 73, pills with breakfast.

Feel okay.

10am Prednisone 20mg fifth day, feeling okay still.

Out to lunch and shopping, feel okay until left side of neck starts hurting in store, then slightly dizzy. Vitamin Magnesium, potassium, calcium all in one pill vitamin.

2:30pm home feeling okay, sweating from outside.

Pretty good afternoon, felt well.

8:30pm, laying down to read, then hopefully sleep.

Will take ½ valium again, as last night.

10:30pm to 2am, fell asleep till 4am. Stayed awake a while, then slept till 6am stayed awake.

9/16/2014 Tuesday

Not great this morning. Hot lying in bed and hissing in right ear, nervous a little and bowel movement right away this morning.

7:30am breakfast and b/p pills

9:15am. another bowel movement and very nervous inwardly. Haven't taken prednisone yet, not due to until 10am. Still hissing in ears.

10am Prednisone 20mg sixth day

Not good this morning, slightly dizzy, very nervous, and not good mentally.

Made smoothie as yesterday, spinach, blueberries, cherries, almond milk. Drank this with prednisone and after.

11:30am slight headache.

1pm having trouble taking in breath, as I sometimes do when lying down at night.

Then sharp pains in left breast, as I've had for years, Angina or Soy in Ensure nutrient drink?

Eating lunch, still have breathing and pain.

2pm now eyes feel fatigued, swollen, tired. I guess from waking up at 4am. This morning.

Fell asleep from 4 to 5pm.

Woke feeling better, but then developed headache.

Dinner 6:30pm. Took Plavix first, then verapamil, and fifteen minutes later coated baby aspirin.

Still feeling tired. Will go to bed 8:30pm.

Slept 11pm until 4am then awake. Off and on sleep then up at 6:30am

9/17/2014 Wednesday

8am b/p 120/80 pulse 86

Breakfast and b/p pills 8:30am

Feeling okay this morning, even took shower.

9:15 prednisone 20mg seventh day

Seeing General Practitioner's assistant at 10am. Feel okay, no wheezing this morning.

GP's assistant asked me more about wheezing, and decided to give me a breathing test, (taking deep breath and blow into a tube). I found when I blew air out of my lungs I wheezed, even though I was not wheezing this morning. I then started to cough. She suggested I take stomach pill Protonix twice a day for reflux, which might be causing the wheezing.

12pm., still felt good.

12:30pm lunch same as last night, left over. Chicken, broccoli, penna with garlic and oil.

Took magnesium, potassium and calcium vitamin after lunch. Taking vitamins on my own hoping they will make me feel better.

2pm still feel okay.

Felt good all day. Around 4:30pm. began to get mentally not right, depressed, maybe? Not really sure. Not really confusion, but scared of this disoriented feeling.

8pm still feeling fine.

Just read stomach pills side effects. May be causing my problems. Been taking it over a year, since I was taken to hospital with pain in med-section. Hospital doctor said could be stomach not heart pain. Interesting. Take a pill to stop burning in stomach and it causes something else if taken long term.

Bed to read around 8:30, 9pm

Good day. Thinking and physically.

Took over the counter Zantec instead of Protonix stomach pill, then ½ Valium around 10:15pm.

Slept well all night, woke once around 2am.

9/18/2014 Thursday
Woke around 6am, feel okay.
b/p 125/80 pulse 63
8am b/p pills Diovan and Metoprolol
10am prednisone 20mg eighth day
Feeling okay except for slight hissing in ear.

11:30am to 12:30pm, Out walking in stores and outside, feeling hard to take breath, short of breath, wheezing.

Not good, came home.

1pm lunch, chicken, penna pasta, broccoli, and ice cream. 2pm Still feeling short of breath sitting down.

4 - 5pm. laid down, fell asleep for few minutes, eyes swollen, and still short of breath.

Had ice tea before eating, thinking, maybe belly filled with fluid retention, tea act as a diuretic. Dinner 6pm, very short of breath, but while eating I noticed I could take a deep breath. What is this? Just like the other night this happened while eating.

Still hissing in ear.

7pm Fell dizzy surge while sitting in chair.

Took blood pressure, 148/76 pulse 78 (high)

8pm, can breathe fine, but belly still blown up.

I'll take Protonix tonight. Didn't take it last night, took Zantec instead, and didn't have stomach burning today.

Bed 8:30pm to read. Protonix 9:15pm then ½ Valium. Slept till 2:30am, then took another ¼ Valium, slept, then awake rest of night.

9/19/2014 Friday

Up at 7:30am, feel okay except for wheezing and congestion in throat/chest.

b/p 117/84 pulse 72

8:30 b/p after breakfast

10am prednisone 20mg ninth day

Nasal drip and congestion this morning, wheezing.

Went to doctor's office, noticed while at office my nasal drip left along with congestion. Was out till 12:30pm. Came home and ate lunch. Within fifteen minutes nasal drip back and started to wheeze again. Is Condo causing congestion?

5pm sweats starting.

Okay tonight, a little antsy, nervous, but not bad.

5pm b/p 106/72 pulse 76

8pm sweats, slightly nervous but not bad. Not tired.

Going to bed around 8:30 to read.

Slept from 10:30pm to 1am. Woke, wide awake, took ½ valium, settled down and fell asleep for maybe an hour, then awake and sleep. Woke around 5:30am not good, hissing in ear, sleeping on my right side, (stroke feeling) mentally not good, pounding in right side of head. Went to bathroom and took b/p (higher than normal) 140's/80's. Laid down trying to relax, drank some Ensure and water and fell asleep.

9/20/2014 Saturday

Woke at 8, b/p 111/74 pulse 69.

8:30 breakfast, then b/p pills, feel okay.

10am Prednisone 20mg day ten last day, then down to fifteen.

11:15am, feeling okay, drinking smoothie, spinach, cherries, blueberries, coconut water, almond milk and sunflower seeds.

2pm lunch, chicken soup.

2:30 magnesium vitamin.

4-5pm fell asleep on couch, woke wheezing and belly blown up.

6:30 dinner, still very blown up, swollen belly and feet and wheezing.

7pm outside air is easier to breathe then inside air at 78 degrees.

Will go to bed around 8:30-9pm. Eyes swollen most of day and feeling tired.

Fell asleep around 11pm then woke at 2am, then woke at 4am very congested, and hard to breathe.

9/21/2014 Sunday

Awake at 4am, congestion and hard to breath. Laid awake, propped up in bed, then fell asleep for a while.

When awake, wheezing, nasal drip. Went to get out of bed, left ankle cramping, foot turning inward.

8am b/p 134/82 pulse 69, blood pressure pills.

Wheezing still and nasal drip.

10am Prednisone 20mg. last day on 20

12pm 111/76 pulse 69

Not great mentally after eating lunch. Seems every time I eat my stomach blows up and I don't feel well mentally. ??

3:15pm still not great mentally, but okay breathing wise. I shut off the air-conditioner auto fan this morning, see if there is a difference in breathing.

5-6pm went out to store in rain, felt better outside of house.

Dinner late, 6:30-7pm. Feel okay, nasal drip, but not bad.

Bed 9pm, read till 10:30pm

Slept till 2am woke, slept till 4:45am then woke and stayed awake for quite a while.

9/22/2014 Monday

Up at 7:15am, soon as walking I started wheezing on outbreath. Feeling slightly nervous. Crazy dreams again last night, this is since prednisone, I think.

b/p 122/84 pulse 72

8am b/p pills

Hissing in ear this morning, 9am.

10am Prednisone 15mg. first day on 15.

Out of the house most of the day, feeling okay, mentally thinking is good.

2:30pm back home after fries, soda, burger, feeling okay.

7:30pm, still okay, other than eyes burning, tired, red. Nasal drip, not as bad as usual. Belly blown up since lunch, burger, salty fries, and dr. pepper.

Sweats at 8pm for the first time today.

Going to bed soon, hissing in ear, eyes burning, and sleepy.

Did good on 15mgs of prednisone today.

Sleep by 10pm, woke in middle of night for bathroom, noticed headache (sinus headache) like before prednisone.

9/23/2014 Tuesday

Woke at 5 then up at 7am. When up started wheezing right away, also slightly dizzy, woozy, feel very congested.

b/p 124/84 pulse 69

8am b/p pills with breakfast

9am could go back to sleep, sleepy, and nasally, left eye still red for three days now. Not great this morning.

10am prednisone on 15 from 20.

Still have congestion, nasal, also still feel slightly dizzy, woozy. Had tea, waffle with prednisone. Tea seemed to clear congested nose.

Ache in right cheek down to upper lip, didn't last a long time.

8pm hard time breathing, not short of breath just hard to take breath.

Went to bed at 8:30pm better lying down.

Protonix at 9pm, then ½ valium at 9:15 then fell asleep. Very tired. Slept till 12midnight, bathroom, then slept till 2am, slept, then awake at 5am, slept, then 7:30am.

9/24/2014 Wednesday

Woke feeling relaxed, not nervous as usual. Slept well last night, even though I woke three times.

When feet on the floor I hear wheezing right away.

8:30 121/79 pulse 67

Breakfast and b/p pills. Hear hissing in right ear.

10am b/p 119/76 pulse 69

Prednisone 15mg third day on 15 down from 20

Out between 11and 12:30 in store, feeling good, very relaxed. Had stomach cramps twice. When home cooked meal and had lunch, sausage, penna, broccoli, olive oil, garlic and onion. Before eating belly bloated (no reason). Back aches from standing up.

1:30pm Ate lunch.

3pm, still hissing in right ear, no other problem

Still feeling relaxed.

4:30 to 5:30 lay in bed reading, resting, back hurt from cooking. Slept maybe 15 minutes.

Feel antsy/nervous when up, ate dinner 6 to 6:30pm still feel antsy. Hissing in ear all day, when up.

But otherwise felt okay today.

Will go to bed around 8:30, 9pm to read.

Fell asleep by 10pm woke at 1:30, then again at 4:30am. Didn't sleep well, sweats.

9/25/2014 Thursday

Didn't sleep well last night and woke very early 4:30am. Woke feeling nervous, teeth clinched, took sip of Ensure, then back to sleep.

8am b/p 121/72 pulse 70

8:30 breakfast and b/p pills

Not great this morning, aching body, hips, legs mostly, and nasal.

10am Prednisone 15mg fourth day

Rheumy today, Bone scan normal. He said, "take 15mg for two weeks then drop 1mg."

4pm feel tired, sleepy

Belly bloated today, laid down from 5-6, fell asleep, woke belly down, then ate dinner, belly up.

Will go to bed around 8:30, 9pm.

Sleep by 10:30pm woke two times.

9/26/2014 Friday

Up 7:30am feel okay. b/p 123/78 pulse 69 Wheezing.

b/p pills at 8:30pm with breakfast.

Burning right nostril this morning, hope it's not like the beginning before on prednisone.

10am prednisone 15mg fifth day

Feeling okay, went out 12:30 to 4pm, didn't eat lunch until 2pm.

Had nuts around 4:30pm, check for headache or auras of eyes, later tonight or tomorrow from nuts.

5:30 okay except for hissing in right ear.

8:45pm, nasal, sneezing, hissing in right ear, eyes feel swollen today (fluid retention), belly blown up.

Going to bed.

Sleep around 10:30, woke at 3am, back to sleep then 7am. Bathroom one time.

9/27/2014 Saturday

Woke feeling okay, slightly tired, stiff and achy.

8:30am b/p low 98/71 pulse 68. Seems funny after having chips (salt) yesterday.

Haven't taken b/p pills yet.

9:45am b/p 121/72 pulse 69

Took b/p pills with food, light headed most of morning.

10:15am Prednisone 15mg sixth day on 15 with food.

Belly blown up after lunch, burger, fries, soda (being I had low b/p this morning I tried to raise it to feel better, less light headed.

Out from 12:30 to 3pm, in stores.

b/p 101/71 pulse 72, old machine, tried new machine and found b/p was 135/78 pulse 70, so will need to get rid of old machine, it's wrong.

6:30pm Plavix, aspirin, verapamil, all within half hour.

Belly still blown up, all day.

Going to be around 8:30 – 9pm

Slept well, up two times 12:30am and 4:30am (cramps in feet, ankles) back from before 20mgs.

9/28/2014 Sunday

7am Woke cramps in feet, stretching, getting out of bed, also not good nervous feeling. Wheezing.

8am new machine 138/80 pulse 71 (don't know if this is right?) will need to buy new blood pressure machine.

8:15am breakfast and b/p pills

Hissing in right ear.

10am prednisone 15mg seventh day.

Achy this morning, hips, back.

Fell asleep at 2:30 on couch, tired, sleepy, belly bloated. Scalp is itching like before prednisone.

7:30pm b/p 129/78 pulse 72 (new blood pressure machine) same make as old one.

Eyes burning, hissing in ear.

Bed 8:30 or 9pm to read. Slept well all night, woke two times 2am and 5:30am.

9/29/2014 Monday
121/78 pulse 79
8:30am b/p pills.

Not good this morning, feeling like stroke feeling.

10:45am prednisone 15mg eighth day

1pm 116/80 pulse 79 before lunch (low b/p) maybe this is why I've felt bad all morning. Belly is blown up.

Spoke to doctor old GP about congestive heart failure. He said my lungs sounded clear, talk with cardiologist on Wednesday for ultra sound.

2:30 still not great. Had pretzels for lunch to make b/p go up.

Low b/p all day, belly blown up, also.

Bed 9pm. Fell asleep around 11pm woke at 1:30 then again at 5:15am.

9/30/2014 Tuesday
Woke rested, but still tired.

8am b/p 121/86 pulse 72

8:30 b/p pills Diovan, ½ metoporal as always.

Lightheaded, even before b/p pills, I think because of low b/p.

10am prednisone 15mg ninth day.

2pm to 4pm out to store, walking.

Came home and fell asleep for an hour, very tired today, belly bloated, and low b/p with new machine.

8:15pm hissing in ear, b/p 120/79 pulse 79.

Going to be shortly.

Slept from 10:30 to 1am, then to 4:45am.

10/1/2014 Wednesday

b/p 120/79 pulse 80

b/p pills 7:45am wheezing right after shower.

9:30 prednisone 15mg tenth day

Cardiologist today, didn't see him saw PA instead. Wants me to have stress test, I said 'no'. Told her about b/p staying low in morning and through-out day, mentioned congestive heart failure and having ultra sound done. She said couldn't do it today, next week. (I'm not happy about this being I am wheezing in the office. She said lungs sounded clear, could be bronchial tubes, upper respiratory problem.

b/p in office was 145/80's (I'm glad it's higher than it has been.)

Told her I was eating salted pretzels in morning to bring b/p up, she didn't like that idea. Said maybe cut Diovan in half. I may try this.

2pm home 119/80 pulse 79 after eating broccoli, penna, sausage, garlic and oil, out at restaurant.

4pm wheezing, in air-conditioned condo

Belly blown up all day. Wheezing.

8:30pm b/p 121/87 pulse 71

Prontonix early, 8:45pm (2 hours after verapamil, may interfere)

Going to bed, fell asleep then woke at 10:30 and took ½ valium.

Woke at 2am heart pounding in head, b/p reads 137/79 on wrist cuff which tells me it's higher. Fell asleep.

10/2/2014 Thursday
Woke 5am, fell back to sleep after crazy dreams, got up at 7:15am.

b/p 124/84 pulse 79. Breakfast and b/p pills
still red bloodshot left eye for week and half.
9:30am prednisone 15mg eleventh day.

11:30 to 2pm out to stores and walking. Feel okay, but at times lightheaded.

b/p 133/79 pulse 72

lunch same as yesterday, leftover, (salted food)

okay afternoon, but lots of hissing and chirping in right ear.

8:45pm going to bed. Chirping in ear, and hissing.

9:30pm protonix
10:15 ½ valium

10/3/2014 Friday
Wheezing when out of bed. Didn't sleep well last night, up a lot, toward morning belly blew up. Didn't bother me last night.

8am b/p 119/89 pulse 79
8:45am Divoan, ½ Metoprolol

Throat very congested with phlegm.

10:15am prednisone 15 twelfth day

Been okay this morning.

Cooked lunch, lentil soup.

2pm almost done eating got nervous feeling throughout body then started getting forehead headache.

3pm still have slight headache. (I did have sunflower butter spread this morning, and two peanut butter crackers) possible migraine? I don't think so.

4:30pm fell asleep for half hour, woke without headache.

Dinner 6:30, soup, two cookies and milk.

Regular pills then 7:30pm Magnesium pill 250mg (new) to relax muscles.

Bed 9pm, protonix.

10/4/2014 Saturday

Woke very early 4am, stayed awake falling in and out of sleep. Out of bed 7am, feel relaxed, not nervous.

b/p 120/89 pulse 68

8:15am b/p pills with breakfast

10am prednisone 15mg thirteen day

2pm lunch, pasta, meatballs, chicken tomato sauce, ice cream. (very little salt in all)

From 3:30pm not feeling well mentally, hissing in ear, not confused, because I know where I am, not disoriented, know the time and place. Very hard to say how I feel when this happens. Not depressed, feeling like nothing, maybe that's the word, nothing. 4pm b/p 125/81 pulse 79 still not well. Too much sugar, (pasta, ice cream) or not enough salt, (sodium) just had three salted pretzels to see if I feel better.

I wish someone could find out what's wrong. Prednisone? Temporal Arteritis? What is it?

At times I wonder if this is the beginnings of dementia or Tia's I may have had in the past due high blood pressure attacks.

5pm magnesium pill, ½ 500.

6pm forehead headache, eating dinner, Plavix, Verapamil, aspirin.

7:30 still have headache.

Bed at 9pm, slept well.

10/5/2014 Sunday

Woke feeling well, not nervous, or anything else. Throat still feels like sandpaper, but that's been for months.

137/85 pulse 69 (feel good, always when b/p is in 130's.

8am b/p pills with breakfast

10am feeling sleepy (b/p pills I guess. b/p now 119/72 pulse 79.

10:15 prednisone 15mg fourteenth day (last on 15)

Now 12:30 getting ready to eat lunch. Windows have been open all morning, cool outside, finally rid of headache.

1:30pm Lunch same as yesterday, pasta, meat, chicken, then ice cream for dessert.

3:30 like yesterday not good mentally, not disoriented or confused, just not right. Craving salt.

4:pm pretzels, and smoothie (coconut water, cherries, blueberries, spinach, and sunflower seeds, raisins.

Magnesium vitamin.

7:30pm feeling tired.

Bed early again tonight probably.

b/p 134/82 pulse 77

Sleep by 10:30, protonix and ½ valium before time.

Woke around 1am, and stayed awake till 4, then slept and woke again at 6, then slept, and woke at 8am.

10/6/2014 Monday

Feeling very tired and heady this morning. I guess because of not enough sleep. Also belly is blown up even before getting out of bed, and feet feel swollen.

8:30 b/p 119/81 pulse 80

8:45 Breakfast and b/p pills

Not good this morning still, heady, hungover, not right mentally. Took shower even though I don't feel well. Always afraid I'm going to lose my balance, fall and break something, or pass out.

10:15 Prednisone 14mg first time on fourteen.

Meeting this morning, women's support group, not good, dizzy, lightheaded.

Went to get up from chair and loss balance due to dizziness/lightheaded. Slight headache.

When home still the same, 1pm.

b/p 140/86 pulse 82 (higher than usual)

Went out to eat burger, fries, soda. (usually I feel better when I eat salt and caffeine soda)

4pm, still not great, but better than I was. Tired though.

Bed 8:30pm to read, fell asleep around 10.

Up once to the bathroom then up at 3am. Still awake at 4:45am and got out of bed to write here.

Just awake, peeing twice since 3am. Belly still bloated, swollen.

Is this because of the lower dose of prednisone to 14?

10/7/2014 Tuesday

8am 124/82 pulse 72

Breakfast and b/p pills

Heady this morning, lack of sleep probably, belly still blown up. Wheezing

10am Prednisone 14mg second day.

Swollen eyes this morning, need sleep.

2pm lunch chicken, string beans, sweet potato, ice cream, green tea. And magnesium, potassium, calcium vitamin (500)

3pm feel just okay, lack of sleep.

4pm b/p 119/76 pulse 80, having chips, nuts, soda.

Hard time breathing today, very short of breath, like belly is into chest, and lungs can't go deep.

6:30 Plavix, verapamil, aspirin which eating dinner, chicken, broccoli, pear, milk, cookie

Very hard breathing while eating, and afterward, belly blown up, but not greatly.

Lowered the temperature to 76 degrees. Noticed I felt better breathing after an hour

9pm bed, easier to breathe lying down, and cooler.

Echo cardio gram tomorrow, check for congestive heart failure.

10/8/2014 Wednesday

Slept well, woke one time at 3am for bathroom, then woke at 7am. Up at 7:15, wheezing, but feel okay.

8am b/p 127/74 pulse 72

Breakfast and b/p pills.

9:30 Prednisone 14mg third day

10am Cardiologist for heart echo. (tech said the results would be on doctor's desk by afternoon)

After walked around stores, feel okay but belly still blown up, left eye bloodshot, now going on almost three weeks, (comes and goes) walking started to feel hard to breathe when it got hotter and more humid.

12:30pm. home, sweating, but feel okay. Haven't eaten lunch yet.

Before lunch oatmeal in water, stir and drink as yesterday.

Lunch, egg, ½ banana, waffle and butter.

2pm bathroom poop, as this morning. (maybe it's the oatmeal from yesterday and today)

2:30 out to store again, walked more. (in store felt spasm in left breast, as I did before prednisone)

4:30pm. home. sat down and got cramping in left foot, I guess from walking more than usual. It finally settled down. Sneezing.

Bed 9pm fell asleep by 10pm, woke one time 3am

10/9/2014 Thursday

Bad nightmare last night, heart beat fast, and sweating, scared, terrified at times.

Woke at 6:30am up at 7:20.

b/p 119/86 pulse 72

8am breakfast and b/p pills.

Feel okay. Eyes slightly swollen.

10:15 prednisone 14mg fourth day, drank pills with oatmeal and water. b/p 124/85 pulse 73.

2 to 3pm lunch, chicken, greens, cucumber salad with olives (salty), ice cream. Magnesium, potassium, and calcium vitamin.

After eating feeling scared, anxious, almost terrified as in my dream last night.

b/p 115/76 pulse 82

Wheezing and forehead headache.

5:30 to 6:15, read on couch falling asleep. Woke heavy headed, and ate dinner. Chicken salad, ½ banana, greens, cookie and milk with pills (Plavix, verapamil, aspirin.

7:30 still feel heavy headed.

9:30 protonix

10:30pm. ½ valium

Slept well, woke one time 3am. Calm.

10/10/2014 Friday

8am breakfast and b/p pills

Bathroom right away this morning after breakfast, maybe the eating raw oatmeal in water for three days is working. Normal movement.

9:30 124/78 pulse 83 (feel okay mostly, only slightly off)

10am prednisone 14 fifth day, with some raw oatmeal and water.

Feel pretty good today, outside of pounding in head.

2pm lunch with magnesium, calcium, and potassium, all in one vitamin.

134/86 pulse 80

5pm fell asleep for half hour. Wheezing.

6:30pm all meds with oatmeal, cheerios, grapes and Ensure. (still pounding in head)

9pm sweats, pounding in head.

b/p 158/92 pulse 70

going to bed.

Protonix 10pm

½ valium 10:30pm sleep.

Woke almost every two hours.

10/11/2014 Saturday
awake at 5am, laid in bed reading.
8am 105/80 pulse 80
Breakfast egg, waffle, ½ banana, bottle of water
9am 102/79 pulse 78
Blood pressure too low, waiting to take b/p pills.
Drink more water, maybe dehydrated.
9:50am b/p 119/79 pulse 75 took blood pressure pills.
10:45am prednisone 14mg sixth day.
Having trouble breathing today, wheezing a lot.
Fell asleep in chair, then laid on couch slept dreaming for hour, maybe. Woke with headache at 2pm, and had lunch, hamburger, ½ banana, grapes, milk and cookie.
Forehead headache most of the day. Went out to store around 4pm. Not good in store, fast heartbeat. Home around 5:30. I did notice breathing better in store, whether it's because the air was colder than home or not. Coming home I turned the air down to 77.
Bad dinner, salami and ham on Italian bread, then ice cream, and Ensure.
Not good, I know. But I'm tired of eating right and feeling lousy. I'd rather eat lousy and feel bad.
Not good mentally either, hissing in right ear. Don't know if b/p is high. I'd rather not take it and fear.

Eyes have been swollen all day, and blurred eyesight, plus the sunlight bothered eyes today, saw green iridescent dots, when eyes closed.

Will go to bed early tonight, didn't sleep well last night, up almost every two hours.

Fell asleep by 9:30. Took protonix

Woke at 12am and took ½ valium

Slept till 6am

10/12/2014 Sunday

b/p 8am 119/80 pulse 72

breakfast no pills yet.

9:30 b/p pills

Aching in right cheek bone, hissing in ear.

10:30am Prednisone 14mg seventh day with food.

Feeling okay this morning.

2pm lunch chicken and salad, ice cream.

Not great mentally and belly starting to blow up after eating food. Always seems to blow up after eating.

3pm magnesium, potassium, calcium vitamin, ½

5pm had ice cream soda, pretzels.

Dinner oatmeal (steal oats, raisins, walnuts) milk and pills 7pm

Sleepy. Going to bed 8:30pm.

10/13/2014 Monday

Up a few times last night, woke at 7:15am

8am b/p 129/90 pulse 72

Breakfast then blood pressure pills. When I looked in the case for b/p pills it was empty. I hope I didn't already take them before, and am now taking them twice. I find it odd that I didn't fill the case with b/p pills last night and filled all others. (not like me)

Feeling lousy this morning, hug over so to speak, black circles under eyes, and bottoms of feet near from feel numb. Belly blown up already even before breakfast. (salt yesterday, chips?)

10am prednisone 14mg eighth day

Feeling bad all morning, took shower feeling shaky. I notice the sweat that comes from me smells different, very bad. (prednisone?)

11am Went to meeting at clubhouse, unable to join in conversation, couldn't think of words to say. Finally around 11:45 started to feel better, joining in conversation, even coming up with my own ideas. Blood pressure? Blood going to brain?

1:15pm before lunch, b/p 142/80 pulse 69 feeling better, able to think correctly.

2pm lunch chicken, ½ apple, drink (spinach, cherries, blueberries) ice cream.

Kind of dull feeling this afternoon, depressed, maybe.

Dinner late 7pm pasta, sausage, broccoli, oil and garlic. (may send the b/p up)

Bed 9pm

10/14/2014 Tuesday

Slept very well last night up one time. And woke feeling well this morning.

8am b/p 125/85 pulse 72
Breakfast and b/p pills
10am Prednisone 14mg ninth day
Feeling good this morning, not swollen, eyes, or belly, or feet. Haven't had that much water.

2:30 Doctor Cardiologist) b/p 145/80 results on Echo. Good heart muscle, only problem (mild) leakage of Mitral Valve. I've had this since heart attack 2011 and two stents inserted.

He wanted to change drug Verapamil but I didn't want to. He doesn't like calcium blockers. (I don't know which drug he wanted me switch to, but also said he studied under the doctor who found Ventricular Tachycardia on me in 1990 at hospital in Fort Lauderdale. (he found it by shocking the different chambers of the heart and when he hit the right ventricle it set off the arrhythmia. He then gave me Verapamil and four or five days later did another Cath test, shocking heart and the arrhythmia didn't happen. So he knew he'd found the right drug to stop my arrhythmia.) I told cardiologist now, "I don't want to stop a drug I've been taking for years."

8pm Good day all around. Just felt good, no effects from prednisone.
9pm hissing in ear first time today.
b/p 115/75 pulse 72
Going to bed. Fell asleep around 10:30pm. Woke two times.

10/15/2014 Wednesday

Bad getting out of bed this morning. Even before I got out of bed I didn't feel right.

6am. Awake. A little worried about Eye doctor appointment today. Feel off, head wise and body, sluggish.

b/p 113/80 pulse 72 waited for blood pressure pills.

7:30am 121/81 pulse 73

Breakfast and b/p pills

Okay but not great, like yesterday. Wheezing, and belly feels swollen.

8:30am Eye doctor's appointment. Feel okay in office. He gave me a good exam and said, "Because you have Giant Cell I want you here every three months. If you have any eye sight problem, like blindness in eye, go directly to hospital."

Stayed out for a few hours, but as time went by I felt worse. 10-10:30 in store really bad, almost falling down from lightheadedness.

11am home, took blood pressure 114/82 pulse 71, very light headed, and this is after taking groceries in from car. So I was using up energy.

11am. Prednisone 14mg tenth day (late by an hour)

12pm. lunch, pieces of rolled up salami and cup coffee. Something to bring b/p up.

12:40pm feel like going to sleep. But won't.

Not good all afternoon.

Lunch/dinner 3pm pork chop, potato, spinach, ice cream.

Feel slightly better, but still tired and light headed.

5:30pm to 6:30pm laid down, and fell asleep.

7pm b/p 124/79 pulse 71 still feel tired.

Pills, verapamil, Plavix, aspirin.

Belly still blown up, wheezing and hard to breathe.

9pm bed

10pm protonix, sleep, then around 3am and took ½ valium.

Slept well.

10/16/2014 Thursday

Woke left ankle and foot swollen.

8am. b/p 121/87 pulse 73

Breakfast then b/p pills

10am prednisone 14mg eleventh day

Fairly good morning.

Made lunch 2pm, soup, beans, carrots, celery, onions, garlic, pasta. dessert ice cream. Then magnesium vitamin.

4:30pm. fell asleep on couch. Vitamin makes me go to sleep an hour or so after. (calcium? Magnesium? Potassium?)

When woke I felt disoriented, confusion, delirium?

Haven't had this in a while. Checked blood pressure 126/84 pulse 71

6:15pm Dinner left over sausage, broccoli, pasta, garlic olive oil. Pills, Plavix, aspirin, verapamil.

Have slight headache today, tenderness in cheek bones, and pain in left side of neck and back of neck since yesterday. I wonder could this be from GCA?

9pm bed to read.

9:30 Zantec instead of Protonix for stomach. Been taking protonix for a long time.

10pm. ½ valium.

10/17/2014 Friday

Slept okay last night, woke around 2am. feeling heart pounding in head.

Everything feels swollen this morning, eyes, hands, feet, belly.

8am 120/81 pulse 69

8:30 breakfast and b/p pills

Not good this morning, lightheaded.

10am Prednisone 14mg twelfth day.

Most of the morning and into afternoon lightheaded, not good mentally, almost like yesterday after sleeping, but not as bad. Left eye seems to be more red again. Eye doctor said it's the aspirin and Plavix. I may skip baby aspirin tonight.

2:30pm after eating lunch, still not great.

4pm feeling tired, yawning.

6pm dinner, chicken salad, hot dog, cookie and Ensure. And pills.

Feeling very, very tired. (fatigue) haven't felt like this since before prednisone started.

7:15pm need to lay down, can't stay awake, exhausted.

Bed, fell asleep right away.

Woke with a start around 10pm, out of it, not aware of time or day.

Read awhile, then took protonix (stomach pill) then ½ hour later ½ valium and fell asleep.

Woke at 2am and stayed awake awhile, then back to sleep, maybe an hour later.

10/18/2014 Saturday

Woke around 6am. Stiff from laying in same position.

Pounding in right ear. Concerned about last night's falling asleep at 7pm. Haven't felt fatigued like that in a long, long time. (thinking, could it be Mini TIA's I had day before when I felt so confused, disoriented. And the day later feel very tired?

8am b/p 124/82 pulse 79

8:30am breakfast and b/p pills

10:30am Prednisone 14mg thirteenth day

Feeling good this morning, even writing, creating, book wise.

Lunch ½ salami sandwich, ½ banana, bean salad, oatmeal cookie.

Feeling mentally good still.

4pm out to food store, feel good, walking around, mentally and physically.

5:15 home, invited company for dinner.

6:30pm ate dinner, chicken, orzo salad, coleslaw, bean salad, biscuit, ice cream, small milk with pills.

8:45pm still okay after cleaning up kitchen from company.

9:30pm protonix then bed to read.

½ valium 10pm sleep

Slept well, crazy dreams. Pounding in head.

10/19/2014 Sunday

Woke, body hurts, hips and back, slight headache.

Wheezing also.

8:30am b/p 122/76 pulse 72

Breakfast 9am Diovan and Metoprolol, (same every morning.)

Not good this morning, tired and cold.

10:30am prednisone 14mg fourteenth day (last day on 14mg)

Spasms in mid-section.

12pm tired and very cold b/p 108/67 pulse 72 just had smoothie (cherries, blueberries, spinach, coconut water trying to drink water to up the blood pressure. Maybe this is why I'm so cold?

Not a good day. Belly blown up, slight forehead headache on the right side.

1:15pm Lunch, chicken, macaroni, coleslaw, biscuit, ice cream. Took magnesium vitamin.

Spasms in back after lunch washing dishes. Laid down around 2:30 and fell asleep. Woke at 5pm. with cramps in right foot, sleepy, and wheezing.

7:43 still not good, wheezing, belly blown up, took a suppository, stool is hard peanuts.

Eyes still feel swollen with slight headache.

9:30pm protonix then bed to read
Fell asleep woke at 1am. Took ½ valium.
Woke two, three times after.

10/20/2014 Monday
Woke around 6am, not great, dry throat, wheezing, nervous inside feeling but yet tired. Drank some Ensure, maybe low sugar from no dinner last night but yogurt and banana.
8am b/p 119/80 pulse 79
Breakfast then b/p pills at 8:45am
10:30am Prednisone 13mg first day on thirteen
Meeting at 11am, out of house till 4pm. Ate lunch out sausage, penna, broccoli, oil and garlic around 2:30pm. Out of house five hours.
Back, hips hurt, and wheezing all day.
But a fairly good day.
Dinner yogurt, mashed pumpkin, nuts, honey.
To bed at 9pm to read.
9:30 protonix fell asleep.
Woke at 1am, took ½ valium
Slept till 5:30am then awake.

10/21/2014 Tuesday
Woke at 5:30am nauseous right hip hurts. Stayed in bed till 7:30am.
b/p 127/85 pulse 72
8:30am breakfast and b/p pills
10:30am Prednisone 13mg second day

Feeling tired, dragging b/p 109/66 pulse 74

Left eye very red as a week ago (may hold aspirin tonight, per eye doctor)

2:30pm lunch, bad. Wendy's, hamburger, fries, and dr. pepper. ½ magnesium vitamin.

Ice cream at home within the hour.

4:30 tired, sleepy. (is it sugar from soda and ice cream?)

6:30pm dinner broccoli, pasta, garlic and olive oil.

Plavix and Verapamil (no aspirin due to red eye)

Tired still 7:30pm b/p 119/82 pulse 73

Head is very hot and sweaty.

Bed 9pm. Protonix 10pm. ½ valium 12midnight.

Awake a lot after 2am.

10/22/2014 Wednesday

Awake a lot last night. Cramping in feet and ankle. Didn't get up till 8am.

Wheezing right away

8:30am. b/p 121/81 pulse 69

Breakfast and b/p pills.

Tired, body aching this morning, hips (right hip).

11am Prednisone 13mg third day on this dose

12:30pm b/p 119/71 pulse 79

1:30 lunch, soup, peach, roll, ice cream.

3pm Magnesium, calcium, and potassium vitamin.

Feel depressed, tired, aching, hips, legs, feet hurt, and back.

Left eye not much better even without aspirin last night.

4:30pm fell asleep for half hour, feel very tired, (sugar? Ice cream?) or magnesium?

Dinner, chicken, greens, cookie and milk. Took aspirin, Plavix and verapamil.

8:30pm tired, eyes feel swollen slightly, belly blown up.

b/p 120/80 pulse 79

8:45pm Going to bed

9:45pm protonix, 11pm ½ valium, slept well.

10/23/2014 Thursday

Woke 8am dreaming crazy. Slept well last night, maybe protonix and valium taken last night.

8:30am 118/79 pulse 78

9am breakfast (cereal, fruit, grapes, ½ banana) then b/p pills

Feel okay this morning.

11am Prednisone 13mg fourth day dose

No lunch to speak of today, Ensure, ½ banana, peanut butter crackers.

Not too great today, belly swollen, also felt slightly dizzy when out walking in store.

Left eye hurts, but not as red. Both eyes feel swollen.

6:15pm Dinner pork chop, sweet potato, broccoli, cookie and milk.

Not a great day, slightly dizzy in store.

Tonight, swelling in legs, feet and ankles, also eyes.

9pm bed.

9:30pm protonix, 9:45pm ½ valium

Bad night, woke at 2am and stayed awake till 5am.

10/24/2014 Friday

Woke feeling very tired, fatigued. Pounding in ears while awake early morning. And hissing.

Up out of bed at 6:20am.

7am b/p 121/87 pulse 72

Breakfast cereal, then b/p pills around 7:15am

Feel very fatigued and aching in hips, (right especially) wheezing. Body was very swollen last night before bed.

Rheumy doctor this morning 9am

Doctor said, stay on 13mg for ten days or two weeks then drop to 12mgs. Said this is a crucial time. Have blood work done in three weeks, see him the end of November.

10:30am Prednisone 13mg fifth day, coffee and donut.

Stayed out, hard walking today, slow and hurting, hips, back, and feet.

1pm lunch half ham sandwich with mozzarella cheese and half an apple, then ice cream.

Today, I feel like I'm dying. I can feel it may be true. I feel something, fatigue, very tired, hissing in ears.

Fell asleep 4 to 5pm on couch, woke with forehead headache. Tested sugar 116, a little high being I ate lunch at 1pm.

B/p 137/81 pulse 74

6pm. Eating dinner, cabbage, casserole with carrots, celery, ground meat, cream sauce (made with mayo). ½ banana and oatmeal cookie and cup of milk, with b/p pills and aspirin.

7pm still have headache and hissing in ears.

9pm protonix and bed. Read for a while then slept, woke at 12midnight took ½ valium

Slept well

10/25/2014 Saturday
Up at 8am feeling good.
b/p 127/84 pulse 72
breakfast and b/p pills at 8:30am
feeling okay, throat raspy. Ache in body, hips.
Cool air outside.

Lunch 1pm ham and cheese ½ sandwich, bean salad, and ice cream.

Nervous this afternoon, no reason.

b/p 119/74 pulse 69 craving salt, had five small pretzels, and three peanut butter crackers and coconut water. Magnesium, potassium, calcium vitamin,

Still later feeling nervous, agitated, laid down and read.

Dinner cabbage casserole, ½ apple, oatmeal cookie.

7:30pm not feeling well mentally, disoriented to time. Feel is should be earlier, just finished eating and taking pills.

b/p 145/89 pulse 79

Not tired, I guess because of the higher blood pressure.

9:30pm still feeling nervous, and hot, hissing in right ear. Going to bed to read.

Taking protonix.

Slept well till 12:30am, then took ½ valium slept till 4:45am, then awake till 6am fell asleep till 7:30am.

10/26/2014 Sunday

7am Glands in neck feel swollen and aching.

8:30am b/p 120/93 pulse 71

Breakfast and pills, Divon and Metoporlol (new, different maker of pills, yesterday also) different look to it.

11am Prednisone 13mgs. Seventh day

Half cheese and ham sandwich and half banana with

Prednisone.

12:30pm to 2pm fell asleep. Very tired, sleepy (crazy dreams)

2:30pm wheezing and short of breath, bad. Haven't had this is a while. Belly blown up, haven't had much to drink this morning.

4pm still short of breath and wheezing. b/p 138/88 pulse 79.

Had green ice tea to drink, peeing a lot after.

Ankles and feet 'not' swollen.

Hissing in ear

5:30 feeling better breathing wise, hissing still in ear. Mid-section still large and swollen.

8pm belly still blown up, dinner 6:30pm steak, ½ baked potato, and bean salad, cookie, and ice cream.

8pm eyes feel swollen, tired, sleepy, hissing in ear, pounding earlier.

Bed soon, very tired. (from yesterday's feeling out of mind around 7:30pm? Mini stroke? Tia?) next day, today, tired?

10/27/2014 Monday

7:30am up feel okay

b/p 120/80 pulse 72

8a.m breakfast

8:45 b/p pills Diovan and ½ Metoprolol (not new the generic)

10:15am. egg, ½ banana, Vitamin D, slice of ham left over smoothie from yesterday (cherries, blue berries, spinach and coconut water)

Not hurting this morning at all? Smoothie yesterday and today, (Vitamin D, or milk magnesium last night) pooped a lot this morning, small pieces filled toilet, twice.

10:15am Prednisone 13mg eight day

11am out to meeting, then to lunch, burger king soda, hamburger and fries, then to eye doctor, then to store. Home around 5pm. Still feeling okay, not hurting as usual. WHY?

7:30pm still okay, a little hyper, as most of the day, but not hurting at all, not fatigued. Is it hyperthyroidism?

All I know is I felt great all day.

Bed around 9pm to read.

9:30 protonix then ½ valium by 10pm lights out.

Slept till 2:30am then bathroom, then up at 4:20am stayed awake for long time. Wide awake, then drifted until 7:15am.

10/28/2014 Tuesday

Out of bed by 7:30am, don't feel as good as yesterday, aching this morning, and slight sweats.

b/p 119/79 pulse 72

Breakfast 8am b/p pills Diovan and old metoprolol until drug store gets in brand name Toprol.

Hissing in ear this morning, and pounding in ear when awake at 5this morning.

10:30am Prednisone 13mg ninth day with boiled egg, ½ banana and drink (spinach, cherries, blueberries and coconut water)

Still aching this morning and hissing in ear.

Lunch chicken, spinach, mashed potato and apple, still not feeling great.

Out from 12 noon till 3:30, hurting back, feet and legs. Hissing in ear.

b/p 120/84 pulse 80

Dinner at 6pm cheerios, seeds and raisins, Ensure, 4 peanut butter crackers. (not hungry) with evening pills.

8pm tired, sleepy, can't stop yawning.

Going to bed shortly.

9pm in bed, didn't even read. Took protonix fell asleep, woke at 12midnight, took ½ valium fell back to sleep. Woke at 5:30am on my right side, head doesn't feel good mentally and physically. Walking to bathroom neck hurts and feels out of place. I twist and turn to feel it crunch back in place, then take some Ensure, thinking maybe low sugar is cause, being I only had cheerios for dinner. Within 20 minutes I feel better and drift off to sleep.

10/29/2014 Wednesday

Woke early as I said above, not good, head wise, mentally and physically.

8:15am. out of bed, very sleepy this morning.

b/p 120/83 pulse 71

9:30 b/p pills with breakfast

Feeling slightly lightheaded, and sleepy

11am Prednisone 13mg tenth day

Not great this morning.

1:30pm lunch Cooked chicken with mushrooms, basil, and mozzarella cheese, carrots, broccoli salad, ice cream. Vitamin D, 2,000.

3pm feel burn in sternum, rib cage, like when I was diagnosed with heart attack. Get this every once in a while. Too full of a stomach, bloated, or heart.

4pm took Tums for burning sternum, ribcage, then fell asleep for an hour.

Woke with headache above forehead, and confusion to the time of day.

6:30 ate dinner, chicken, carrots, bean salad, oatmeal cookie, milk/ensure and b/p pills, Plavix, aspirin.

7pm b/p 115/82 pulse 72 still have headache

Eyes swollen today, most of day.

Don't like waking up from sleep (whether it's day or not) being disoriented, confused.

8pm b/p 141/89 pulse 75 an hour later higher b/p

Still feel not good, headache, swollen eyes, belly blown up, right upper above eye brow aches. Not good mentally. Possibly nervous.

9:15pm. going to bed to read.

Read till 10 took protonix then woke at 3am and took ½ valium. Crazy dreams about death.

10/30/2014 Thursday

Woke at 6am and stayed awake, got up at 7:15am.

b/p 119/81 pulse 69

8:30 breakfast then took b/p pills Diovan and new metoprolol.

Eyes feel swollen.

11am Prednisone 13mg eleventh day.

12:30 to 2:30pm Burger King meal, then beach tried walking a little in sand, very hard, breathless, but beautiful sight. Left foot and ankle swollen.

Ice cream.

6pm dinner steak and greens, 2 oatmeal cookies and milk with pills.

b/p 133/84 pulse 72 hot on top of head and sweats.

8pm hissing in ear, eyes swollen, not so tired, but soon to bed, to read.

9pm bed, 9:30 protonix, sleep by 10:30pm.

Woke at 1:30am ½ Valium, awake for a while, back to sleep, awake at 5:45am.

10/31/2014 Friday

8:30am 126/83 pulse 66

Breakfast and b/p pills Divon and Toprol (brand name) first time.

11:20am Prednisone 13mg twelfth day

b/p 129/87 pulse 67 slightly dizzy

12:15pm cramping in lower belly, like going to get diarrhea, but didn't, just dark stool from yesterday's juice (spinach, cherries, blueberries)

1:15pm 113/77 pulse 69

Lunch, pasta, chicken, sausage, beef. Ice cream afterward.

3:30pm pounding in right ear, head area, as at night or early morning hours in bed. b/p 129/81 pulse 72

5:15pm headache b/p 124/80 pulse 70

6:30pm pills, verapamil, Plavix, aspirin with dinner.

Deaf in right ear. Hearing came back then pounding in ear. (may need wax cleaned out)

Nervous tonight, also during daytime. No reason, just nervous.

Bed 9pm, protonix 9:30 sleep by 10pm

Woke at 1:30 ½ valium slept till 5:15am

11/1/2014 Saturday

Woke very early, then fell back to sleep.

8am b/p 124/84 pulse 68

Blood sugar reads 90 (felt a little odd this morning)

Breakfast and b/p pills after breakfast 8:30am 2nd day of Toprol ½ pill (Brand name)

11am Prednisone 13mg thirteenth day

Feeling mad, depressed, sad, something along those lines today.

Had ice cream after lunch, 1:30pm – 2pm

3pm feeling bad, eyes swollen, nervous, but yet depressed, hissing in right ear. Checked blood sugar 148, high (range on test says 112-149. Had some yogurt for protein.

Something just not right, sugar, maybe, slight headache, and very depressed, mad, etc. even hard to speak right when neighbor came for visit.

4:30pm. laid down to read, get my mind off myself. Laid there looking at the ceiling instead.

6pm sugar 137 still fairly high. Had chicken, egg, and toast with nut butter, hot chocolate without sugar.

6:30pm pills and dinner.

Bed at 9pm to read. Read till 10 protonix, slept.

1am ½ valium slept and woke up, slept and woke.

11/2/2014 Sunday

7:30am b/p 133/84 pulse 70

8:15am Breakfast and b/p pills Diovan and Toprol (3rd day brand Toprol)

Chilly again today outside. Windows open, easier to breathe, but still wheeze on out breath. But better with windows open and cool air instead of air-conditioner on at 78 degrees.

10am prednisone 13mg fourteenth day

11am to 12pm fell asleep.

Wheezing worse when I got up. Apparently laying down made it worse. WHAT IS IT? Asthma? Congestive heart failure? What?

1:30pm lunch, chicken and tomato sauce, pasta, ice cream. Wheezing still. Eyes swollen again.

Wheezing all day.

6:30pm dinner oatmeal and Ensure, with pills.

8:30pm hot, and peeing a lot after dinner. (no reason) Going to bed to read, feeling tired.

Asleep by 10pm protonix at 9:30pm valium ½ at 1am. When I woke up. Bad dreams.

11/3/2014 Monday

Woke around 5:30am after a bad dream, and headache, sipped Ensure and back to sleep. Up at 7:30am.

b/p 120/82 pulse 78

8am breakfast and b/p pills.

Still slight headache and feeling down, maybe the bad dream.

10am Prednisone 13mg fifteenth day.

11am to 5pm out, meeting at club house, then lunch, doctor, and then store. Long day, hurting, aching in hips since this morning, and left side of neck. Interesting I have not been wheezing while I'm out of the condo. Why?

Came home at 5pm. As soon as home and started sneezing, Now at 7pm I've been wheezing for the last hour. What is causing it? There is tile on the floor, hardly any drapery, couches have been cleaned, What is causing the wheezing?

7pm Hissing also has started in right ear.

8pm milk magnesia for bathroom, tomorrow.

8pm to bed, tired. No reading, fell asleep, woke at

10:30pm took protonix, woke at 2am took ½ valium.

11/4/2014 Tuesday

Up at 6:30am, bathroom, bowel movement from milk magnesia last night, tiny pieces of stool as big as a thumb nail (like always) filled the bowl.

b/p 120/82 pulse 79

7:30 breakfast cheerios, ½ banana, grapes, (made juice, spinach, cherries and blueberries.

8am b/p pills Diovan and Toprol

Sleepy around 10am but not hurting as much as this morning.

b/p 106/78 pulse 79

11am Prednisone 13mg sixteenth day

Not bad today, lower back aches, and feet, especially walking in store or standing cooking.

3pm lunch/dinner broccoli, sausage, pasta, oil and garlic. Good. Ice cream afterward.

6:30pm cereal, milk and oatmeal cookie, with pills.

9pm going to bed. Belly feels so much better after moving bowels 3 times.

Going to bed.

11/5/2014 Wednesday

Slept well.

7am up, leaning over sink washing face, wheezing, right away

7:3am. b/p 108/80 pulse 72

8am breakfast

8:20am b/p pills Diovan and Toprol

Coughing this morning, feel congestion.

10:15am Prednisone 13mg seventeenth day

Took shower and felt worse in shower breathing wise, harder to breathe, and coughing, wheezing. I thought a hot shower would help, but it didn't and made it worse.

2pm to 5pm out hard to breath no matter where I am. Weather is overcast and raining off and on. In air-condition office hard to breathe also, coughing with wheeze on the out breath.

7pm still wheezing, now hissing in right ear.

Achy all day in hips.

Eyes feel swollen, feet swollen and ankles.

Going to bed early, around 8pm

Sleep by 9 after protonix.

Woke at 11:30pm took ½ valium back to sleep. Woke two times there after.

No breathing problems.

11/6/2014 Thursday
Woke early 5:30am out of bed by 6:30.
7:30am. b/p 133/78 pulse 73
Breakfast and b/p pills Diovan and Toprol
8:30 starting to wheeze.
10:15 prednisone 12mg first day on twelve
b/p 115/78 pulse 66

Had yogurt, ½ banana, and drink (spinach, blueberries, cherries, coconut water)

Not wheezing bad, like yesterday, very light today.

Feeling depressed as yesterday, or down, so to speak. Thinking about my life and health, being poor, and being ill. Where do I go, and what do I do?

Started coughing after lunch, drink went down wrong pipe. Coughed then stared whistling wheeze.

Out from 2:30pm till 4:30pm stopped at pulmonary doctor's office and made first time appointment. Can't get in until December. Eye doctor recommended I go. Do I have pulmonary disease?

Then to store, tried walking around in store to get my breathing going. I almost feel better in store then at condo. Something in Condo causing wheezing?

6:15pm dinner pork chop, sweet potato, squash, oatmeal cookie and milk, with pills (verapamil, Plavix, baby aspirin).

For some reason better breathing after eating. Something to do with stomach being full? Yet, I hiccup most of the time after eating. Thinking about taking protonix (stomach pill) in day time instead of right before sleep at night. A thought.

8pm still feeling okay breathing wise. Will go to bed within the hour and read for a while.

Protonix at 8:30pm, read a while then sleep. Woke at 12:30am took ½ valium back to sleep. Woke two more times. Not a good sleep.

11/7/2014 Friday

7:15am. feeling nervous, heart pounding in head.

b/p 127/78 pulse 72

8am breakfast then b/p pills Diovan and Toprol

Hissing in right ear.

Bending down putting shoes on started to whistle wheeze.

10:15am. Prednisone 12mg, second day

Not bad rest of day.

Plumber came and used a cleaner. Feeling hard to breathe. I opened windows and air-condoner on.

3:30pm to 4:30 fell asleep.

Woke with hiccups.

5pm took Protonix 40mg (stomach pill I usually take at bed time) see if this makes a difference in my breathing after dinner, when I usually wheeze.

6pm dinner, Plavix.

6:30 verapamil b/p pill, 7pm baby aspirin.

7:30pm. very tired, fatigued, little sleep last night, but also could be protonix early instead of at bed time.

Hiccupping after dinner even though I took protonix, before dinner.

7:45pm going to bed.

Lights out by 9:15pm fell asleep. Woke at 11:30pm. took ½ valium. Fell back to sleep woke at 4:45am and stayed awake until 6am, then back to sleep.

11/8/2014 Saturday

Awake at 7:15am.

b/p 128/84 pulse 80

8:30 b/p meds. Diovan and Toprol

Eyes feel swollen, pain in hips, and hard moving rest of body. Tried mopping floor and found it hard to bend and move.

10am Prednisone 12mg third day. I wonder Prednisone is causing down feeling, or depression?

Okay morning. Worked my books.

4pm starting to wheeze, door has been open to outside for past two hours, but also I took protonix at 5pm yesterday. Hiccupping a little.

4pm b/p 135/79 pulse 82

4pm took protonix, early, instead of waiting till bed time.

Bathroom department is still the same, hard small balls, peas, so to speak.

6:15pm dinner, pills Plavix, aspirin, verapamil.

To bed 9:30pm. Read till 10, then sleep. Woke at 1:30am pounding in head, fast heartbeat. Took ½ valium, fell asleep, woke next time at 5:45am.

11/9/2014 Sunday
Not great this morning, eyes swollen, wheezing as soon as out of bed, throat feels gritty, coated with chalk, but isn't. maybe from milk magnesium last night.
7:15 b/p 119/68 pulse 72
8am breakfast
8:20am b/p pills
Bathroom, small tiny stools, as usual.
10am Prednisone 12mg fourth day
Feeling okay today, stressed working on new book. Going well, can think okay. Haven't been able to write in a long time. Possibly the prednisone reduction?
Was great up until around 3:30pm when neighbor came to chat during lunch. I had hamburger, chips, and soda. Felt good, but then after talking a lot about writing and doing my books, I began to lose my train of thought. Just too excited about my writing, I guess. I could feel my face hot, possible blood pressure up. But haven't taken it.
6:30pm took Plavix with dinner, 20 minutes later Verapamil, then 7:15pm baby aspirin.
Tired from working all day on book, and using eyes a lot. Will go to bed around 8:30.
10:30 ½ valium going to sleep.

Woke at 1am, then back to sleep. Woke at 5:30am with cramps in ankles and feet, wheezing, pounding in head.

11/10/2014 Monday

Woke at 5:30am with stiff cramping in ankles and feet, pounding in head, then wheezing. Nervous feeling. Laid awake and read in bed until light came up.

6:45am b/p 137/86 pulse 73

7:30am. breakfast and b/p pills Diovan and Toprol

Feeling okay, slightly hung-over from valium,(I think)

10:15 Prednisone 12mg fifth day

Shower, feel worse in the hot shower, wheezing. Harder to breath. Breathing through mouth.

11am went to meeting, feel tired, but okay mentally, can think okay.

Then out to store and shopping. Sweating a lot while in store, feeling like blood pressure is high, red face, and out of breath when walking fast.

Out until 3pm. Total of four hours.

When home had ice cream to cool down, it seems to work, and breathing is better.

Dinner, chicken, collard greens, grapes, milk, cookie.

b/p 135/80 pulse 79

Bed at 9pm lights off at 9:45. Slept till 1am took ¼ valium, slept till 3am took another ¼ valium.

11/11/2014 Tuesday

When woke at 6:30am. I felt pretty good, had a good sleep outside of waking for bathroom two times. Breathing is good, not wheezing.

7:45am. breakfast

b/p 137/85 pulse 80 took Diovan and Toprol ½

Feel okay at 9:30am. Brain seems awake, alive. Not aching a lot, different room and bed last night (hard) maybe that's why not aching much.

10am Prednisone 12mg sixth day.

12:20pm. lunch chicken salad, pretzels, grapes, ice cream.

Feeling okay today.

Started wheezing late afternoon.

3:30pm Protonix with peanut butter crackers and milk.

Worked on writing today. Had spasm in left upper rib cage and had to give up working.

Fell asleep around 5am lying on bed. Still wheezing.

6:15pm dinner, chicken, broccoli, squash in chicken broth, two oatmeal cookies and milk, with pills Verapamil first, Plavix, then aspirin last.

9pm to bed and read, till 9:45. Woke at 2am took ½ valium and fell back to sleep.

11/12/2014 Wednesday

Woke around 6:30am. out of bed at 7am.

Didn't take b/p, for some reason I knew it was normal.

Breakfast 8am after that Diovan and Toprol.

Whistle in chest, then wheeze but feeling okay.

10am Prednisone 12mg seventh day

Lunch, (no lunch really) had tomato, basil, mozzarella cheese with olive oil. Two cups of ice cream afterward.

Neighbor visit from 2:30 to 4pm. Didn't feel good while visiting.

4:15pm. Ensure, thinking my brain doesn't feel well, hard to think straight, came up with the right words, while at neighbors. Hard remembering what happened years ago, when taking care of friend with Alzheimer's.

Now drinking water. Hate this feeling of losing one's self. One's mind. That is what it feels like. I met another neighbor in the lobby, getting mail. He also took care of an Alzheimer's person, and I have the feeling he also is losing his mind. I feel sorry for him. Do others feel sorry for me when I'm like this? Do they know I'm like this? Or do I hide it well?

Plus it could all be from not eating correctly at lunch time. Too much sugar.

6pm dinner, eggs and bacon, milk and two oatmeal cookies.

6:15pm verapamil, fifteen minutes later Plavix, then baby aspirin.

Tired tonight/today. Better mentally after eating dinner. 9pm bed to read, fell asleep 10pm.

11/13/2014 Thursday

Slept well last night, took ½ valium at 1am when up for bathroom. Fell back to sleep then woke at 6am.

7am b/p 145/91 pulse 70, same as last night before bed.

Took b/p again ten minutes later 128/77 pulse 70 ate breakfast at 8am then took b/p pills.

During eating breakfast and after I notice diarrhea cramps in lower stomach. Went to bathroom, dark stool as yesterday, soft, not little peas as usual. Interesting.

Been to the bathroom three times with cramps and loose stool.

10:30am Prednisone 12mg eighth day

Been drinking bottled water since yesterday morning. I wonder if bowel movements are from this and not drinking tap/fridge filtered water?

Going for blood work today from Neurologist and Rheumy.

12:30 blood work, still not good mentally, almost worse. Haven't eaten lunch yet.

1pm Lunch out, pasta, broccoli, sausage, oil and garlic, one garlic roll. Still don't feel better mentally after eating. Onto store, not good in store, hard to breathe. Taking deep breaths, and sweating a lot.

3:30pm home, still not good mentally, and thought, maybe have a UTI, which effects my brains thinking, brain fog, out of it feeling. Will take pee test next.

3:45pm protonix 40mg

4pm ice cream and one piece of chocolate.

5pm UTI test shows lots of blood in urine, and infection level dark green. Possible UTI. Maybe doctor tomorrow will check this.

Still not good mentally and getting chills again.

6pm dinner. Same as lunch plus two oatmeal cookies and milk. Took Verapamil first, then fifteen minutes later Plavix, then fifteen minutes later baby aspirin. Instead of taking three meds together.

8pm Just got off the phone with an old friend I found it hard coming up with right words to say and my face very red when I looked in mirror. I guess blood pressure is up, but I don't feel like taking it right now.

9pm bed, read for half hour then to sleep.

11/14/2014 Friday

Woke at 4 this morning, but fell back to sleep after ½ an hour. Slept till 7am. Feel still not great. Temp 98.1 usually around 97.5. Maybe UTI increasing temp. Also slight headache.

8am. b/p 140/95 pulse 80, high for this time morning breakfast then b/p pills.

10am prednisone 12mg 9th day

b/p still high 145/90 pulse 80

Not wheezing until I took shower at 11am. Hard breathing in shower and wheezing afterward.

b/p running higher, 150/92 pulse 80, feel hot today, and red faced.

Have company, maybe that's why b/p up.

9pm 150/96 pulse 88 (high) red faced. Going to bed.

½ valium at 10pm then woke at 3am and took another ½ valium.

11/15/2014 Saturday

Woke around 6am, and laid in bed. b/p still high, face red. b/p 168/96 pulse 107, having skipped beats.

Breakfast

8:20 another ½ Toprol hoping b/p will come down, feeling slight dizziness.

Now wheezing.

10:20am b/p 159/96 pulse 80

10:30am Prednisone 12mg tenth day

11am started wheezing and coughing.

12:30pm 145/86 pulse 80

2pm pounding in head/left ear.

2:30 143/86 pulse 80.

4:25 feel b/p up and afraid to take it.

6pm dinner cereal, banana, and grapes along with two oatmeal cookies and milk

Took verapamil first, then Plavix, then aspirin, all within a half hour

8:15pm b/p 159/92 pulse 79

Going to bed to read.

Will take protonix around 9:30pm then ½ valium. Hope I sleep tonight without high b/p.

Woke at 3:30am and took another ½ valium, but didn't fall asleep. Bad forehead headache.

11/16/2014 Sunday

Woke at 3:30am and stayed awake, with a forehead headache

6:15am b/p 175/96 pulse 98

Breakfast and b/p pills, Diovan and ½ Toprol.

8:15am 142/86 pulse 81

Prednisone 13mgs. Instead of 12 today due to forehead headache. Afraid of Giant Cell Arteritis damage.

8:30am laying down, still bad headache

10am still headache, waffle and Ensure second drink today.

b/p 159/94 pulse 93 took ½ Toprol

hissing in ear, and headache still.

b/p high most of day, finally rid of headache maybe because I took another Toprol.

5:30pm pills verapamil, Plavix, aspirin.

143/97 pulse 92 slight headache and shaking today.

8:30pm going to bed shortly, tired. Been up since 3:30am.

Protonix around 9pm and fell asleep, then ½ valium. Slept till 3:30am (seems to be the bewitching hour) stayed awake then fell asleep till 7am.

11/17/2014 Monday

Up around 8am. not good.

b/p 148/90 pulse 80

Have something to eat then b/p pills.

Coughing and wheezing this morning.

10:30 Prednisone 13mgs, second day on thirteen.

b/p 147/88 pulse 92 other ½ of Toprol.

Dizzy and off balance.

4pm b/p 151/86 pulse 89

6 - 6:30pm dinner, soup, milk and chocolate cookie with pills, verapamil, Plavix, aspirin.

7:30pm b/p 169/94 pulse 91

Going to bed early, read then sleep.

Took protonix around 9:15pm, sleep around 10:30pm. Woke at 3:30am. took ½ valium.

11/18/2014 Tuesday

Woke around 7am, tired, coughing, left eye blood shot.

8am. 156/100 pulse 86

Coughing a lot.

Breakfast and b/p meds, Diovan and ½ Toprol

10am Prednisone 13mg. third day on thirteen.

An alright day, better than on 12mgs of prednisone.

b/p high again, 150/80's and pulse high

Bed early, 9pm, protonix, then ¼ valium

woke at 11:30pm, then again at 2am, then again at 5:30am. Tired.

11/19/2014 Wednesday

Up at 6:30am, took shower, tests at neurologist office, EMG test for nerves and muscles, bottom part of body.

7am b/p pills Diovan and Toprol ½

Didn't take another ½ as I've been doing these past few days due to very high b/p. I decided not to take it today.

9:30am, prednisone 12mg. 1st day back to 12mgs.

Testing around 10am, lasted till 11:45am. Testing nerves and muscles in legs and feet, interesting test, I saw a difference in the left leg, foot versus the right leg and foot. Next appointment in Jan. 2, 2015.

Had ham sandwich for lunch, and grapes.

Later around 3pm b/p 137/75 pulse 91.

Ice cream, cookies and piece of chocolate.

At 4pm I couldn't stay awake, falling asleep in chair. Went to bed and quickly fell asleep. Slept till 5pm, Woke with front top of head and forehead aching. Also nose feels like sinus problem.

When I woke I was totally out of it. I looked at the time next to my bed and found I was not within the time, day, or anything else that was going on. Totally disconnected. Could not bring my mind back. All I thought was Dementia. Then remembered the sugar I had had before the sleepiness started. Could it be sugar? Diabetic? Or possibly due to the prednisone I've been taking now for eight months.

6pm dinner turkey hamburger, grapes, Ensure with pills, Plavix, Verapamil, baby aspirin.

Now 7pm. sweating a lot. Hot on top of head, and forehead headache also pain on top of head, and pulse pain on right temple side of head. Nose also running clear liquid. Not feeling right mentally, scares me very much. I think if I was alone, I would have called 911. Good I have a roommate.

Will probably stay up longer tonight, afraid to go to sleep, and wake like after 5pm nap.

9:30pm protonix, in bed reading.

Woke around 2am, took ½ valium fell back to sleep.

Woke around 7am. Slept well.

11/20/2014 Thursday
8am b/p 135/94 pulse 88
Breakfast
8:30am. Diovan and Toprol
10am Prednisone 12mg 2nd day back on twelve

Rheumy doctor today, see him again in a month. Make an appointment with Endocrinologist and stay on twelve mgs of Prednisone unless I feel really bad, then up it to 13mgs.

3pm Lunch chicken salad, grapes, two cookies and smoothie, spinach, cherries, blue berries, coconut water.

6:20pmDinner, broccoli, chicken, pasta, oil and garlic. Plavix, verapamil, aspirin.

Lower back hurting a lot.

Sweating a lot, very hot.

Bed, 9pm, protonix 9:30, ½ valium 10pm

Slept well, until 2:30am., woke, no valium, fell back to sleep.

11/22/2014 Saturday

6am. Woke not good, nervous, seeing colored line in eyes when closed for a second, slight sick to my stomach.

7am. Breakfast then Divon and Toprol

10am. Prednisone 12mgs

Dressed then laid in bed. Not good this morning.

Air-conditioning on all night. Coughing a lot and bad wheezing as soon as I wake. I opened window in my room, and could breathe better.

Sunday

Not good took Prednisone 12mgs.

But later around 3pm took another 1mgs to make it 13mgs total.

Later in evening not good.

Monday 11/24/2014

Not good at all.

Took prednisone 12mgs later in day got a bad dizzy surge/vertigo feeling, first time in a while. No control over my body.

Also high blood pressure 150/90

Later in evening feeling better.

Have straight lines in eye sight, and possible migraine, light one. Also hissing in ear, right side.

Bed by 9pm

Prednisone 9:30pm

½ valium 10pm

Slept well.

Tuesday 11/25/2014

8:30 b/p meds with breakfast

Feeling okay, slight hissing in ears/head

9:30am Prednisone 12mgs (I want to get off this drug) I've developed red dots, like a rash over my body, first on arms, but then see it on belly and legs.

Not bad day.

Got sleepy around 4pm fell asleep till 5pm, felt rested.

6:15pm. dinner, oatmeal, and key lime pie with milk. Felt slightly disoriented to time and place. No brain, thinking wise. Then forehead headache.

Sill at 7:45pm. I still have forehead headache, mostly on the right side of head as before the prednisone. Sinus headache I complained about for months, that no one could find.

Went to bed at 9:30pm took protonix, read till 10:30 and took ½ valium.

Woke at some time feeling right side of neck hurting, and mentally out of it. Fell back to sleep.

Crazy dreams. Woke again around 6:30am, feeling right side of neck still hurting, and mentally not good.

11/26/2014 Wednesday

Up early, b/p 140/86 pulse 81

Ate breakfast and took meds, Diovan and Toprol

10am Prednisone 12mgs and Ensure

Right back side of neck still hurting this morning, really since Monday, when I leaned on my right side. Funny, because the left side doesn't hurting anymore.

Lower back hurts a lot especially cooking in kitchen.

Just had lunch, potato soup and ice cream.

Headache all day, mostly on forehead, right side head.

Dinner same as lunch potato soup.

Went to bed early, headache all day, and wanted to lay down due to lower back hurting.

Read in bed, protonix around 9pm then 1/2 valium

9:45 sleep.

Woke around 3am stomach bothering me, right side of stomach/belly fells hard, yet swollen. Fell back to sleep. Woke again at 5:30am. stomach still upset, nausea.

11/27/2014 Thursday

Woke still not good stomach wise, upset, hard belly, swollen. Also back of mouth taste is bad.

Out of bed by 8am.

97.4 temperature

b/p 135/87 pulse 81

breakfast then pills Diovan and Toprol ½

lower right side of belly/intestines making sounds.

10:30am prednisone 12mgs.

Stomach felt better after eating breakfast.

Had lunch about 3pm, large meal for me. Chicken, potato's, spinach, cranberry salad, ice cream.

Very full, Thanksgiving dinner.

6pm yogurt with nightly pills.

Mentally very good today, even did some writing.

Left foot and leg very swollen, and bottoms of both feet numb up front, under toes, and right in back of toes.

8:40pm. going to bed. May have small snack before bed.

11/28/2014 Friday

Bad night last night, up every 2-3 hours, hard to breathe when laying on right side. This has happened a few times in the last couple days, I've noticed.

Woke this morning, tired, and swollen, belly, feet and eyes.

b/p 137/82 pulse 80

8am b/p/ pills with breakfast

Bathroom not good, small stools as usual, peanut size, brown with white spots in it, as usual. Only move bowels when taking milk magnesia.

Pounding in head, last night also.

Feet feeling numb early this morning. Were very swollen yesterday and last night, even top of foot.

10:30 prednisone 12mg (been three weeks now). Up a day or two when I had bad headache.

11:30am. liquid suppository, then pooped maybe 10 balls size of large marbles.

Left foot still bruised, two toes, side of foot, upper foot swollen, right foot side bruised, also swollen but not like left foot. Both ankles swollen, and red/purple in color. Back of both legs behind knee bruised in circle form. This all started maybe four days ago, getting worse and worse. Had EMG test Wednesday November 19th, Eight days ago. Maybe the feet and leg problems are from the test?

Very tired today, sleepy after lunch. Tried to lay down at 2:30pm, but had company visit.

By 3:45pm I was back laying on my bed, reading, and falling asleep. Very fatigued.

Slept from 4 to 5pm, got up watched TV for half an hour then ate dinner and took Verapamil, Plavix, and aspirin, within half hour.

Now it's 8:15pm and I will be going to bed soon.

Bed around 9pm protonix and ½ valium.

Slept fairly well, woke three times, but fell back to sleep.

11/29/2014 Saturday

Woke around 6am fell back to sleep till 7:30, got out of bed at 7:45.

I felt I had high b/p from the wrist cuff so took Diovan and Toprol with breakfast at 8:30am.

Felt better before b/p pills then after.

10am Prednisone 11mgs first time this morning down from 12.

Very good day. Got a lot done working on writing a book. Worked all morning, into the afternoon. Ate lunch around 1pm two pieces of pizza, and two chocolate candies. Worked more on my book.

Laid down around 4pm to rest my eyes, hoping to fall asleep.

Neighbor rang bell. Neighbor is moving and wanted to say goodbye. Talked till 5:30pm. I began to have a terrible headache along with not being able to think right mentally. Words wouldn't come that I wanted to say. Searching for words. I hate that feeling, plus I felt my blood pressure was high.

Neighbor finally left and I fixed my dinner.

Took blood pressure for the heck of it. 144/81 pulse 80. I wonder what it was while neighbor was here.

Dinner around 6pm turkey burger, spinach, mashed potato.

9pm going to bed. To read.

9:15pm. protonix. 9:45pm. ½ valium then sleep.

11/30/2014 Sunday

Woke off and on during the night, especially 4am, 6am, 6:30am., then at 7am. I didn't want to get out of bed. Fell back to sleep and woke at 8am and got up. Wheezing right away.

Breakfast around 8:30am. b/p 127/89 pulse 80

took b/p pills 8:45am

10:45 Prednisone 11mgs, second day

Felt so good yesterday, but feel bad today. Hard to breathe, breathing fast, dry cough. Not wheezing.

Big difference from yesterday morning.

Mentally worked on my writing a short time, but not good physically. Lower back hurting bad, while I was cooking, maybe twenty minutes. Had to lie down on bed to straighten my back out.

Dinner around 5:30pm., started to get headache front of head, right side mostly. GCA?

Mentally not good, thinking off. Scared. Watching television. High whistle in right ear when breathing out. Short sound, I thought the sound was coming from outside but it's within my head. This happens at times when I lie down at night to sleep.

Took suppository, feeling have to go to bathroom all day, but nothing. This morning two or three tiny hard balls with white around them. Tonight another ten to fifteen hard small balls.

8pm still headache, but not as bad as before. Hissing in right ear.

12/1/2014 Monday

Slept little last night, due to people moving in complex, but then proceeded to wake up every two hours. Finally awake at 6am. got up.

b/p pills 8:30am. after breakfast. Took shower and went to bathroom, still not good after taking milk magnesium last night. (something wrong in bowel)

10:30am. Prednisone 11mgs third day.

Went to club house meeting, feeling good.

Out till 3:30pm. then to store.

Felt good all day, lower back hurt after walking. But other than that, feel good.

7:30pm 120/80 pulse 79

7:30pm hissing in right ear.

No headache today, even had pecan nuts.

Bed early tonight due to little sleep last night, maybe around 8:30pm

12/2/2014 Tuesday
Up late, 7:45, feeling tired, and aching.
All right mentally, but body aches and feels tired.
8:30pm b/p 105/68 pulse 79
Breakfast, b/p still low, no pills yet.
9am, still low p/b after having G2 and bottle of water, figure I'm dehydrated.
10am b/p 119/82 pulse 81 took b/p pills finally.
Not feeling as achy, trying to drink fluid.
11:20am. Prednisone 11mgs 4th day
1pm lunch, chicken soup and roll, water.
General Practitioner
b/p 118/70's belly is blown up.
Doctor didn't like my left leg and left foot, sent me down stairs to Imagining department. Looking for blood clot in leg. They did imaging on left leg, and ultrasound Tec said she didn't see any clots, and doctor will read it.
(So I wait.)
5:30 to 6:30pm dinner and pills, Plavix first, then almost half hour later Verapamil with food, then aspirin fifteen minutes later.
b/p 128/84 pulse 81 (amazing it's stayed low all day) possible because I took first b/p meds at 10am?
Bed around 7:30pm to read. Other pills around 8:45pm, then sleep.

Slept well, except for waking a few times.

12/3/2014 Wednesday
Woke early, but stayed in bed.
Put support hose on left leg before getting dressed.
Whistling wheeze in lungs while lying in bed, after waking.
b/p 117/86 pulse 80
8:45am breakfast then pills, Diovan and Toprol ½ like always.
Feel okay, eyes feel swollen.
10:30 Prednisone 11mgs 5th day
Lay in bed for a while this morning, then around lunch time resting left leg on hassock wearing support hose.
I can feel swelling or movement under the hose, in back left side of left leg.
Also looks like right leg and foot are swelling.
Mentally not great.
3pm laying down in bed to reduce swelling.
Did some writing while sitting in bed today. I see the left leg is not as swollen when up. As soon as I sit down it starts to tingle.
8pm now, and I have my left foot on hassock, but I feel tingling in foot and leg, also in right foot. Numbness on bottom of foot.
Laying down in bed soon. Hissing in ear.
8pm b/p 141/83 pulse 79

Going to bed to read.
Pills around 9pm both Protonix and ½ valium
Fell asleep right away.

12/4/2014 Thursday
5:30am woke and couldn't breathe, felt I was drowning, under water, gasping for air. Very hard time breathing, then scared because of it.
6am up b/p 155/99 pulse 81
Still not able to breathe and wheezing once my feet hit the floor.
6:30 breakfast and b/p pills Diovan and Troprol
7:30am to foot doctor, cut nails and looked at left foot which was not swollen as the last days. Told him about neuropathy, Neuro Doctor, normal for my age.
I like the way he informed me the way the body works: "plumbing, electric, skin, and bones, that's it." Looks like something wrong with your plumbing. As in congestive heart failure, or something else because it isn't pumping blood through the system.

10:am Prednisone 11mgs sixth day
Saw ARNP pulmonary doctor. Waited over an hour in the office, and found breathing got easier, was it because of the prednisone I'd taken?
Doctor sent me to hospital for CTscan of lungs, and also wants breathing test done, which will be done next week.

I think I was concerned of clots in lungs, don't know if CT shows congestive heart failure. But that's the way I felt this morning, drowning.

Was out from 7:30am till 3pm leg did not swell as bad as days prior, but did when I came home and sat in chair. Slept between 5 and 6pm.

Woke with bad chills. Changed clothes to warmer ones, then ate dinner.

Right after dinner I started sweating, hot chocolate maybe, but then I started getting chills again.

Pain still in right groin off and on.

7:30pm b/p 144/82 pulse 80

Hissing in right ear, with heat coming up my neck to my head.

Pray I do not get the breathing problem like this morning again.

9pm in bed, wheezing whistle, then stopped and fell asleep right away, woke one time, slept till 8am.

12/5/2014 Friday
Wheezing soon as feet on floor.
b/p 120/80 pulse 79
breakfast cheerios, half banana, milk.
Pills Diovan and Toprol half pill 25mgs.
Left leg slightly swollen, I guess because of little water to drink yesterday.
Sleepy this morning after b/p pills
10:45 Prednisone 11mgs seventh day
Lunch sausage, broccoli, olive oil and garlic.

Went out to store, hard breathing when outside, humid and warm, short of breath.

Home, laid down for a while, left leg and foot swelling went down slightly. Going to bed at 9pm.

12/6/2014 Saturday

Slept well last night, ¼ valium.

Breathing not good this morning, congestion sort of.

8am b/p 122/80 pulse 79

Breakfast then b/p pills Diovan and Toprol ½

10am Prednisone 10mgs first day on 10mg (hold off if I'm not good take the extra 1mg later.)

3pm. Finding it hard to breathe today, in my room with window open, or in living with air-conditioner on.

Belly feels swollen, left foot and leg still swollen.

For some reason I felt better around 5pm, no real reason, maybe food has gone from stomach? A thought? But then why do I wake in the middle of the night unable to breathe? So that doesn't make sense.

7:15 now, and still feeling okay breathing wise, just finished dinner, cereal, with raisins, and pecans and bottled water with pills.

9pm bed to read awhile. Protonix then ½ valium, woke one time 2am. Up at 7am.

12/7/2014 Sunday

Woke around 7am notice wheeze or hard to breath. When up feel I'm not getting full breath of air. Went outside breathed in deep and started coughing. Did this a few times, breathe deep and blow out.

8am 123/83 pulse 79

Breakfast then Diovan and Toprol ½ 25mgs

10am Prednisone 10mgs, second day of ten

Bad day.

Headache around 5pm, hissing in ear. b/p 128/90 pulse 81.

Dinner around 6:15, took pills with meal, verapamil first, fifteen minutes later Plavix, then 10 minutes later aspirin.

7:30 headache is better. Eyes still feel swollen all day.

Whistling wheeze. Breathing not good all day.

Bed early to read. Went to bed 9pm read for a while, then took protonix 9:30, and quarter valium twenty minutes later.

Had trouble breathing when lying down flatter, so propped myself up before I fell asleep. Woke two times.

12/8/2014 Monday

Woke around 7am got up. Breathing not bad, no phlegm in throat, dry throat.

b/p 124/80 pulse 79

breakfast then Diovan and Toprol half pill

10am Prednisone 10mgs third day.

Hard breathing again. Fatigued, tired, sleepy, b/p pills, I'm sure.

Meeting at 11am at club house. I found it easier to breath then at condo. Cleaning lady came today, using cleansers.

Out again to store. Still okay when out walking breathing. Home at 3pm, had ice cream and pecans.

Will see how it is when home a while, breathing wise.

Dinner around 6:15pm, along with pills, verapamil first, fifteen minutes later Plavix, then aspirin.

Bed early tonight, a little tired, but I'm still able to breathe, and I wrote a little today. Good day.

12/9/2014 Tuesday

Had problem at 4am, Vtack. Haven't had attack in a long time. Fast, irregular heart. b/p high. Took ¼ valium, and settled down.

8am b/p 121/80 pulse 78

Breakfast then Diovan and Toprol

10:30am Prednisone 10mgs, fourth day

1pm breathing test at hospital.

Found it interesting because I had wheezing this morning, especially coming out of shower. Had wheezing during test. Breathing in deep breaths ached behind my breasts. Breathing out I had wheeze and cough afterward. Then tech gave me inhaler to use for few minutes. After that I noticed I could take deep breaths, no wheezing. Lungs felt bigger. Still after the test walking in store I could walk faster without being out of breath, and talking I wasn't out of breath. The only thing I noticed my nose kept running and felt head congestion like I had before the prednisone, sinus infection. I wonder? Asthma?

Now 4pm and still able to breathe good. b/p 119/80 pulse 81 (low for this time of day, but I haven't had much to drink today.

Good rest of evening.

8:30pm No protonix tonight, ¼ valium, slept fairly well, breathing good.

12/10/2014 Wednesday

Woke around 6:30 breathing still good, can take deep breath. Slight wheeze.

8:30am b/p 116/80 pulse 80 (will wait to take b/p pills)

9:30 b/p 128/84 pulse 79, Diovan and Toprol with food.

11am Prednisone 10mg fifth day

Feel okay this morning, left foot, ankle, and leg swollen, more now that I am up. Back of both legs behind knees hurt from the ESR test done on November 19, I called Neurologist's office to relay this.

Neurologist called back, saying swelling and bruising could not be caused by ESR test. Go to your General Practitioner.

I called GP and have an appointment tomorrow 9am. The ultra sound done on the left leg was negative for blood clots.

So what is causing swelling in left foot, ankle and leg? And why do backs of both knees hurt, like black and blue, bruises?

Got tired around 11:30am laid down to read and fell asleep. Seems like every time I lay down I fall asleep. Woke around 1:30pm. ate lunch/dinner around 3:30pm have forehead headache, pounding in head and ears and wheezing again.

5pm still have forehead headache.

Left foot, ankle, and leg swollen.

9:30 protonix, okay night.

12/11/2014 Thursday

Up at 7am, shower, hard to breathe in shower.

Wheeze slight.

b/p 117/79 pulse 80

8am breakfast then b/p pills

9am GP's office, different doctor, b/p 144/80's, weight 203.

Doctor said walk a lot for swollen foot and leg. Gave me script for inhaler for wheezing and breathing, and I need a bone scan, Lucent Lesion on T5 vertebral body. Also lucent lesion in T11. Will make appointment at Hospital for tests.

10:30am Prednisone 10mg sixth day

12pm home.

Felt good all afternoon. Had lunch/dinner at 1:30 steak, baked potato, greens, milk, ice cream.

Feel good, very alert, and thinking right mentally.

Got tired around 4pm, laid down to read and fell asleep, woke at 6pm.

Had yogurt, chocolate pudding, cookie and Ensure.

Took Plavix first, then aspirin, then Verapamil around 7:15pm.

Will 'not' take protonix tonight.

9pm, going to bed, tired, sleepy. Been a long day since 6 this morning.

No protonix, took ¼ valium at 10pm, then to sleep. Woke at 1:30am, took other ¼ valium, slept till 5:30am, stayed awake.

12/12/2014 Friday

Woke early, slept well.

Out of bed around 7am. Moved bowels, right away, three times. I wonder, is it because I didn't take Protonix (stomach pill) last night?

Breakfast cereal, banana and grapes.

b/p 138/84 pulse 80 too pill Diovan and Toprol ½

10:15am Prednisone 10mgs seventh day

1pm Lunch, ham sandwich, milk, then out.

Feeling very tired today, fatigued, legs feel tired, and shaky, along with right hand and arm.

3:30pm blood work for Rheumy, SED rate.

4:30 home extremely tired, ate burger, fries, and little soda, then ice cream, hoping to get some energy.

b/p 134/81 pulse 74

Just very, very tired. I'm dying, I can feel it. Muscles hurt/ache and feel totally depleted, worn out, from nothing.

5:30pm Plavix, aspirin twenty minutes later. Took Verapamil around 6pm

Going to bed 8:10pm. Protonix, Read and fell asleep woke at 1am took ¼ valium

12/13/2014 Saturday

Woke off and on last night, woke at 8am and got up.

b/p 120/80 pulse 79

breakfast 9am took Diovan and Toprol.

11am Prednisone 10 mgs eighth day

11am 107/79 pulse 69

Temperature 96.8, feel very cold, tired and sleepy.

1pm lunch egg salad on slice bread, ½ apple, and hot chocolate to warm me. I'm so cold.

Legs not good, feel weak to walk. Have support hose on left leg due to swelling. Put it on this morning before walking around.

2pm starting to warm up. Blood pressure must be rising.

6pm cereal for dinner.

Not a good day, legs weak. No walking today.

No protonix at bedtime. ½ valium. Woke one time.

12/14/2014 Sunday

Slept well last night. Woke around 6am back to sleep, then up at 7:30am.

8am b/p 120/80 pulse 79

Breakfast 8:30 with b/p pills Diovan and Toprol ½

Put support hose on both legs. Left leg and foot are still swelling, especially as day goes on. I notice foot hurts on the outside top.

10:30am Prednisone 10mg ninth day

Okay this morning, later on harder to breathe.

Out at 1:30pm hard breathing.

Lunch/dinner 3pm meat, sauerkraut, onions. After eating harder to breathe in. Belly feels like it's in my chest, very bloated.

5:30pm. sleepy, right after eating.

b/p 120/80 pulse 79.

Wheezing on the out breath today.

6:30pm. Plavix and aspirin

7pm Verapamil

Peanut butter crackers for dinner. Still very bloated.

Protonix at night

12/15/2014 Monday

Not a great day, but not bad.

135/80 pulse 72

10:15am Prednisone 10mgs tenth day

Stood in kitchen for maybe an hour, back hurt badly, had to lie down.

Friend came to visit, nice surprise, haven't seen her in many years.

Protonix at night, regurgitation after dinner, chicken soup.

Bed by 8pm, fell asleep right away, woke at 12:30am nervous, took ½ valium went back to sleep, slept most of night till 5am.

12/16/2014 Tuesday

Woke not great stomach, even though I took protonix last night. Again regurgitation, hope I don't have blockage. Bowels still small balls even after taking milk magnesia before bed time.

8:45am. b/p pills with breakfast

Not feeling good belly wise. And pounding in head.

10:30am Prednisone 10mgs eleventh day

Out before lunch, felt okay in store, but still out of breath. I tried walking fast hoping to get circulation going in left leg and foot (both still swollen since EMG Nov. 16)

Not bad when home. Chicken salad for lunch and half apple.

Tired around 4pm, fell asleep off and on till 6pm (I'm told my breathing is making me tired)

6:30pm. to 7pm. pills, verapamil first, Plavix, aspirin.

Bed around 8:30pm. Sleep around 10pm woke at 3am and stayed awake quite some time.

12/17/2014 Wednesday

8:30am b/p 124/90 pulse 74

b/p pills while eating breakfast.

10:20am Prednisone 10mgs, eleventh day

At Rheumy's office b/p 145/80

Doctor said two more days on 10mgs then down to 9mgs. as long as no head pain.

Middle of night I tried sleeping on my right side, but noticed I can't breathe in and wheeze on the out breath (rib cage I guess) when I lay on my left side I'm able to breathe okay, better then right side.

Better breathing outside then in condo. I'm going to have to try staying out of condo for a few days, motel, maybe and see how breathing is. Then I will know it's either the condo affecting my breathing or not.

Out all day 10am to 4pm.

Now at 5:20pm. I feel tired and will eat dinner soon, probably an egg and waffle, and grapes.

12/18/2014 Thursday

7:45am b/p 127/89 pulse

Breakfast then Diovan and Toprol ½

Wheezing right away this morning

10am Prednisone 10mg eleventh day.

Out from 8:30am till 12:30pm. While out hurting muscles and cramping in left rib cage under breast.

Lunch/dinner broccoli, sausage, pasta, oil and garlic.

6:30pm inward chills. While eating dinner.

8:30pm. to bed. 138/90 pulse 70 wheezing more today, air-conditioning on most of the day.

Protonix, slept well.

12/19/2014 Friday
8:45am 122/79 pulse 80 (just out of shower)
Wheezing, hard to breathe in shower.
Breakfast and pills Divovan and Toprol
10:20am Prednisone 9mgs first day
Still swollen left leg and foot, have support hose on.

Windows open this morning, better breathing without air-conditioning.

Out around 1pm wheezing, and hard to breathe. Don't know if it was the shower this morning.

Had a headache today.

8pm. still headache and hissing in right ear. I'm sure my blood pressure is up, but I'm not taking it. I'm going to bed and reading a book, to get my mind off possibly being homelessness and where I'm going. If roommate decides to move, I have no choice.

9:30pm Protonix, then ¼ valium, 2:30am ¼ valium still awake. I'm letting my problems effect my sleeping. I have to stop that. I thought I had learned, but I guess I have to relearn.

12/20/2014 Saturday
Sleepless night, up at 8am, out of bed 8:45am. Breakfast at 9am, then b/p pills. Didn't take b/p I'm sure it's high thinking about being homeless again.

10:45am Prednisone 9mgs second day.

Tired.

1:30pm lunch/dinner, penna, sausage, broccoli, oil and garlic.

3:30pm fell into a deep sleep, when I woke 4pm and looked at clock I'd lost all track of what day it is and time. Confusion. Blank brain. Scared, I got up fast for the bathroom, trying to remember what day it is. This lasted for quite a while and then came down with a bad headache, above the forehead, on top of head.

All day headache on top of head above forehead.

Took 1mg of Prednisone 5pm. Thinking maybe it was because I had dropped a dose. Thinking it could be Giant Cell Arteritis back.

Wheezing all day.

8pm b/p 120/80 pulse 80

Still bad headache, going to bed to read.

Protonix and fell asleep, woke at 11 taking ¼ valium, then again 2am ¼ valium. Woke every two hours, possible prednisone taking it late.

12/21/2014 Sunday
8am b/p127/83 pulse 73
Breakfast and pills, Diovan and Toprol
Hissing in right ear.
10:30am Prednisone 9mgs, first day again.
Feeling okay today.

Black and blue mark on top of right foot, similar to the way left foot had month ago. WHAT is THIS? Have a lump, as if I bumped it. (I didn't) I get these on arms, and legs at times. I mentioned it to Rheumy, but he didn't think it important.

7:30pm after eating dinner have hissing in right ear.

Feeling tired, but not bad, eyes feel tired, but I've been working writing today and reading a lot.

12/22/2014 Monday

Middle of night woke with pounding in right side of head. Feet hurt, both of them, went to bathroom, then drank Ensure and took valium 1:30am. Back to sleep.

8:45am b/p 120/80 pulse 79

Breakfast then Diovan and Toprol

Wheezing this morning and afternoon, except when I went to meeting. I noticed the wheezing stopped, and felt okay.

10:20am Prednisone 9mgs. Second day.

1pm lunch, still okay breathing wise, but belly is very blown up, fluid I think.

Both feet hurt and still have black and blue mark on top of right foot.

Went to store and walked around forty-five minutes, just for exercise. Feet, ankles and lower part of legs not good. Red on legs and warm to touch.

5-6pm fell asleep few minutes, woke with chills while eating dinner.

7:30pm still feet and ankles hurt, lower legs hot to touch, odd, because they're usually cold.

Bed early tonight

12/23/2014 Tuesday
Woke 8am up,
b/p 124/80 pulse 79
breakfast and pills Diovan and Toprol
Swollen and hurting right ankle, and foot, top still black and blue.

Called and made appointment for 4pm with doctor taking over for GP.

Both ankles and feet swollen even when I get out of bed in the morning now.

10:45am prednisone 9mgs third day

Right foot not good today, hard to move in morning, but better as the day went on.

5pm saw new doctor taking over for GP, liked him. Old fashion doctor.

He said EMG test did not cause bruises on my feet or swelling. He suggested taking diuretic for three days, if the feet, ankles and legs go down, that means I'm retaining water and no blood clot. He also said if blood pressure goes down below 100 call him. But Christmas is in two days, mostly everyone is closed, so don't know what to do? I'll try pill tomorrow and see what happens.

6:30 to 7pm Plavix first, then verapamil, then aspirin.

Hissing in right ear.

It's 8pm now, and I'm going to bed.

Laid in bed, started to read, then fell asleep. Woke at 9:30pm took protonix and ¼ valium. Woke one time after.

12/24/2014 Wednesday
Put my feet on the floor this morning and they both hurt, feel like the bones of my feet are on the floor, no flesh supporting them.
b/p 113/78 pulse 75
9am breakfast then b/p pills Diovan and Toprol
Not taking diuretic yet, b/p too low still.
Prednisone 8mgs around 11am first day.
Then took 1mgs of Prednisone at 1:30pm. because head felt odd. Total 9mgs forth day.
8:30pm Bed to read and fell asleep.
Protonix then woke at 1am to thunder storm, and took ½ valium, stayed awake for an hour, then to sleep. Feet and right ankle hurts.

12/25/2014 Thursday
Woke feet hurt and swollen, right foot and ankle hurt a lot.
8:30 b/p 120/79 pulse 79
b/p pills Diovan and Toprol with breakfast.
Cold this morning.
11:15am Prednisone 8mgs first time.
Will take extra if needed later.
Didn't feel great today, slight headache later on, don't know if it's weather related or prednisone related. Pounding in head/right ear.
Feet swollen, especially the right foot.

3pm ½ diuretic because feet swollen.

Fell asleep on couch around 4:30pm not great mentally in afternoon.

b/p 6pm 140/84 pulse 79

dinner/cereal, took Plavix, verapamil, aspirin within half hour period.

8pm feel heady, in forehead, right above nose. 9pm156/85 pulse 72.

Bed early. Protonix 9pm, slept till 1am, ¼ valium slept till 6am.

12/26/2014 Friday

Woke feeling okay, feet still swollen, but don't hurt as much. Right foot, ankle, leg seems worse then left.

7am. b/p 130/85 pulse 79

Breakfast and b/p pills Diovan and Toprol

10am diuretic ½.

Feel okay except for slight lightheaded, even before diuretic.

10:30am b/p 120/80 pulse 79

11am Prednisone 9mgs 8th day back up, because eye and headache problems.

4pm b/p 108/72 pulse 75

7pm 114/75 pulse took Plavix and aspirin not verapamil, b/p too low.

Feet, ankles, and right legs swollen, right one hurts most, also developed two bruises on inside of foot.

8pm Verapamil.

9pm 121/65 pulse 73

Bed. Took over the counter stomach pill instead of protonix because taken verapamil late.

Woke around 4:30am very confused to where I am. Lay there trying to get my brain back. Could it be fluid buildup in body causes these setbacks in thinking every once in a while? Or is it Prednisone? Or something else?

12/27/2014 Saturday

Woke around 7am didn't get up until 8am.

b/p 123/75 pulse 65

Weighed myself 198lbs.

Having coconut water, every day, breakfast and b/p pills Diovan and Toprol

9:45am hissing in hear

10:30am Prednisone 9mgs 9th day

11:30am diuretic ½ third day for feet, ankles, legs.

Feet, ankles and legs (right leg) a problem all day.

b/p not high all day.

Bed at 9pm, took protonix slept, then woke at 12midnight took ¼ valium.

12/28/2014 Sunday

8am feet swollen and back of right leg hurts.

b/p 119/79 pulse 79

Breakfast then Diovan and Toprol

10am diuretic ½

11:15 Prednisone 9mgs 10th day.
b/p 127/82 pulse 79
Sleepy.
Headache later on in day over forehead.
b/p low most of day in 120's
6:30pm Verapamil then Plavix, then aspirin 20 minutes later.
Still headache.
Swollen feet, ankles and legs all day.
Notice after eating I wheeze, or when I lay down.
To bed early, feel tired from not much sleep last night. 9:30pm protonix

12/29/2014 Monday
Woke four times last night, just kept waking up.
8am b/p 127/82 pulse 80
Breakfast and b/p pills Diovan and Toprol
Feeling not bad.
10am ½ diuretic
11:30am prednisone 8mgs first time
Feet, ankles swollen all day, not hurting though.
3pm went to store to walk around. Shoes are not fitting too tight due to swollen feet.
Walking in store I found little out of breath, and feet began to hurt, but I walked any way about half an hour for exercise.
6pm dinner and pills, verapamil, Plavix, then aspirin, forty-five minutes in all.
7pm Going to lay down early tonight because feet swollen.

Doctor's office tomorrow.
Protonix. Bed, and sleep by 9:30pm.

12/30/2014 Tuesday
Woke unable to breathe, laying on my right side. I notice I cannot sleep on my right side and breathe right. Went into shower, took a warm, not hot shower, and came out wheezing and coughing.
When out I was tired and out of breath.
b/p 144/86 pulse 80
Used puffer, one time, instead of two which it says on the box.
Noticed I could breathe better, take deeper breaths, but still wheezed. I also noticed my heart beats fast.
8:30am 120/80 pulse 79
Breakfast and pills Diovan and Toprol
10am feeling better, breathing wise and otherwise. Except hissing in right ear.
Feet swollen, but do not hurt. Ankle on right foot hurts and up from ankle.
10am Prednisone 8mgs, second day
Wheezing on the out breath all day.
GP doctor late afternoon. Says, I have a heart murmur, keep taking Lasix and feet look better. I think so too. Take the puffer for wheezing, couple times a day if needed. Sending me for blood work, and Ctscan of abdomen checking for mass.
9pm going to bed. Hissing in ears. Protonix.

Sleep around 10:30pm, slept till 12:45am took ¼ valium back to sleep, woke at 5am stayed awake.

12/31/2014 Wednesday
Woke feet swollen.
8:30 b/p 120/80 pulse 79 pills, diovan and Toprol
Not good mentally, thinking wise.
10am diuretic ½ 20mgs of Lasix generic.
11am Prednisone 8mgs third day
Swollen feet, ankle, and legs today, worse then yesterday, also spasms in rib cage, left side.
Headache later in day, possibly from peanut butter crackers.
9pm 141/83 pulse 80 protonix.
Bed around 10:30pm read for a while then slept till 12 midnight took ¼ valium, slept and woke at 6am.

1/1/2015 Thursday (Happy New Year, ha.)
Woke up with pounding in ear, but feel okay.
8am 120/80 pulse 79
Diuretic ½ Lasix
8:30 am breakfast
Took b/p pills Toprol and Diovan
9:30am b/p 113/69 pulse 79 (low) hissing in ear, lightheaded, sleepy.
11am Prednisone 8mgs fourth day
3-4pm. fell asleep. Woke up wheezing
Hissing and pounding in ear/head after eating dinner.

5pm b/p 129/80 pulse 79 feet, ankles still swollen, especially as the day goes on.

Used puffer, albuterol, one puff. Stopped the out breath wheeze.

6-7pm. verapamil, Plavix, aspirin.

Bed 8:30pm to read, protonix at 9pm then fell asleep.

Woke around 1am took ¼ valium. Fell back to sleep.

1/2/2015 Friday

Woke early 6:45am stayed in bed. When up pounding in right ear/head like yesterday

8am b/p 133/82 pulse 79

Took diuretic ½ Lasix

8:30 breakfast oatmeal and walnuts, raisins and ½ banana.

b/p pills Diovan and Toprol ½

10:30am Prednisone 8mgs fifth day

I have been diagnosed with Asthma and COPD by lung doctor.

Now 1/18/2015 still feel not good, coughing and wheezing day and night. No fever like last week.

B/p has been okay, in fact low.

1/19/2015 Monday

Didn't sleep last night.

6a.m. b/p high. 150/80 on wrist cuff.

Took ½ banana and b/p pills Diovan and Toprol ½

Feeling not good this morning.

5pm first meal, spaghetti, mushroom, chicken, salad, Plavix, aspirin. 5:30pm, cookie, milk and Verapamil.

Feeling better tonight. Will go to bed early. Feet, ankles, and legs still swollen from November's EMG test.

1/20/2015 Tuesday

Slept well last night, first in a while. Woke at 3a.m. from 9:30pm.

Up at 7am. 145/87 pulse 79

Breakfast and pills Diovan and Toprol ½

10:15am Prednisone 8mg twenty-second day

Feeling better after diagnosed with Flu, still cough off and on. No wheezing yesterday, and so far today no wheezing.

Sharp pain/ache under right breast, rib cage, around to back.? Could be muscle pull from coughing so much from Flu.

Amazed I haven't lost weight, being I haven't been eating due to illness. First I ate was last night, starting to have appetite.

6:30pm b/p up again, 145/87

Took Plavix at 5:30pm with food, then Verapamil, then aspirin at 6pm

Feeling bad today, heady and mentally not good. Legs, ankles, feet swollen like every day since November. It started with the left foot.

Nervous and scared tonight. Why? I don't know.

Same old, same old, afraid of being homeless again, afraid of illness again. I have to do something with the rest of my life. I can't go on depending on roommate for a roof over my head. She is ill now, and I shouldn't depend on her. I can't take care of her and myself.
9pm, Scared.

1/21/2015 Wednesday
8am 135/85 pulse 76
Breakfast then Diovan and Toprol ½
Right side under breast still hurts/aches.
10am Prednisone 8mgs.
Not a great day. Feeling slight vertigo this morning, and bad mentally.
5:30 Plavix, verapamil and aspirin with food.
8pm feel okay, still cold then hot.
Bed soon.

1/22/2015 Thursday
Awake a lot last night, sweats, every two hours.
Up at 7am.
b/p 127/84 pulse 78
7:45 breakfast and b/p pills Diovan and Toprol ½
Still right back, side and front hurts/aches. Put a brace on to see if it helps.
10am Prednisone 8mgs 27th day

Not great mentally today.

Fell asleep 3-5pm. on couch and woke disoriented, scared. Feeling ache on right side of forehead and jaw. GCA?

5:30 – 6pm pills Plavix, verapamil, aspirin with food.

Not good tonight, depressed over the way I feel physically and mentally, tired. Bed at 9:30pm.

1/23/2015 Friday

No wheezing, a few days now. Right side, back, belly hurts/aches still all week. Hoping pulled muscle from coughing from Flu.

8am Low b/p this morning. 113/74 pulse 78

Breakfast oatmeal

9:30am 119/79 pulse 80

Diovan and Toprol ½ (late)

Feel like I have a brain this morning, I'm even writing.

10:45am Prednisone 7mgs. first day.

Not bad, feeling today. Laid down from 2-4pm. slept little, but rested body.

6-6:30 pills, Plavix, verapamil, aspirin with half sandwich, macaroni salad, and smoothie, greens, cherries and blueberries.

Hissing in ears.

Bed early tonight.

Awake a lot.

1/24/2015 Saturday
8 a.m. b/p 110/80 pulse 72 low
8:30am breakfast 122/82 pulse 80
8:45a.m. Divon and Toprol ½
Feel okay
10:30a.m. Prednisone 7mgs. Second day
Felt good all day, until 8pm. Started to feel Nashua, throwing up feeling, not good. Had egg, half of a pear and carrot for dinner. Half Ensure.
Slept fairly well, woke a number of times, sweating.

1/25/2015 Sunday
Woke at 6am stayed in bed.
Up at 7:15am
8am b/p 107/85 pulse 71
Breakfast oatmeal, raisins, banana
9:15 pills Diovan and Toprol ½
Wheezing this morning, first in a week or more.
10:30am Prednisone 7mgs third day
Felt pretty good all day.
Bed by 8:30pm read for an hour then took protonix. Awake off and on.

1/26/2015 Monday
Woke at 6am didn't get out of bed until 7.
8am b/p 129/80 pulse 79
Breakfast and pills Diovan and Toprol ½
Feel okay, still pain, ache in left side front back, two weeks now.
10:30am Prednisone 7mgs fourth day.

b/p 100/66 pulse 72 drinking more, coconut water and G2.

b/p low all day, headache, fell asleep around 4:30pm. a few minutes.

Took Plavix and aspirin at 6 while eating dinner.

7:30pm taking Verapamil now.

b/p 99/57 pulse 67 had some salted pretzels and water.

8:45pm b/p finally up 135/79 pulse 69

Bed early tonight to read.

1/27/2015 Tuesday

8am 108/76 pulse 72

Breakfast oatmeal trying to eat it everyday.

No b/p pills yet b/p too low

10am b/p 129/79 pulse 72

B/P pills Diovan and Toprol ½

11pm Prednisone 7mgs fifth day

Slightly dizzy in shower low b/p

Out from 11:30 – 4pm

Blood work for Rheumy and food shopping.

Right side, back, and front hurts still now going on two weeks. Have brace on, still hurts when standing.

6pm b/p 135/76 pulse 62

Dinner and Plavix, Verapamil, aspirin

Felt okay today except for pain in right side.

Sleep 10:30pm. Woke a number of times.

1/28/2015 Wednesday

8am 122/83 pulse 79
Breakfast oatmeal
8:45am b/p pills Diovan and Toprol ½
Doctor said take 7mgs for ten more days then lower to 6mgs. B/p in his office 120/82 weight 201lbs
10:30 Prednisone 7mgs sixth day
Out from 9:30am to 12:30pm doctor then store. Side hurts, especially when home after being upright.
3pm b/p 116/70 pulse 70 craving salt, had potato chips.
5pm 119/75 pulse 70, headache
6pm dinner and pills Plavix, verapamil, aspirin.
7:15pm. tired. b/p 99/66 and wheezing. Haven't been wheezing. I do wonder if it's low blood pressure when I wheeze.
Went to bed, side hurts. Read till 9 then took protonix, then sleep, wheezing lightly.

1/29/2015 Thursday
Woke last night at 12midnight and stayed awake a while. Off and on sleep most of the night. Awake at 4:30am. Read till 6am then fell asleep till 7.
Wheezing lightly
8:30am 117/77 pulse 72
Breakfast
9am b/p 107/73 pulse 80 (no pills yet, b/p too low.
9:30am b/p 118/79 pulse 73
Pills Diovan and Toprol ½

11:30 Prednisone 7mgs Seventh day
Lunch out 1pm. sausage, broccoli, penna garlic and oil. (usually makes my blood pressure go up.
Came home 3:30pm
b/p 113/76 pulse 72
9pm b/p 120/80 pulse 69
While reading I almost feel like I'm getting eye Nystagmus (eyes going back and forth)
Bad headache. Tylenol then at 10pm protonix.
Wheezing laying down.
Woke a lot during the night.

1/30/2015 Friday
Slightly dizzy this morning. Feels like vertigo.
Wheezing also
8:30am 112/81 pulse 72
Breakfast still dizzy
9:30am. 140/80 pulse 70
Diovan and Toprol ½
Still head problem
10:45am. b/p 126/77 pulse 66
11am Prednisone 8mgs. First, back to 8 because of head feeling. (see what happens rest of day)
Head got better, no headache.
8pm b/p 120/80 pulse 72
Hissing in ear and feeling tense.
Rested from 5-6pm.
Going to be to read 8:45pm
Protonix at 9pm sleep at 10pm
Woke at 3am, stayed awake till 5am.

1/31/2015 Saturday
Up around 8am
8:30 b/p 126/81 pulse 79
Breakfast oatmeal
Diovan and Toprol ½
Right side still hurts.
Feet, ankles, legs not swollen like last night.
11am Prednisone 8mgs second day back again.
Feel slight headache this morning.
Lunch around 1pm.
Later, not good at all. Headache and head tenderness, on top of head, pain when pressed.
Hissing in ear later.
Aching behind left breast after eating dinner.
Feel PMR/GCA are back. I don't want to go up on Prednisone.
Wheezing today, lying down this morning.
Bed at 9:30pm read awhile then sleep before 10.
Woke around 11pm disoriented, fast heartbeat, panic. b/p 168/95 pulse 122. Skipped beats. Feels like my Vtack attacks.
Took ½ valium, tried to relax and breathe. Went down within fifteen minutes. 122/78 pulse 72.

2/1/2015 Sunday
Slept well after last night's Vtak attack. Woke around 5am.
8am 120/79 pulse 79

8:45 breakfast and took pills Diovan and Toprol ½

Slight headache 10am

b/p 114/70 pulse 69

11am Prednisone back to 7mgs. First day again. Two days on 8. I'll see what happens. Later if I'm feeling bad I'll take 1mgs. (headache gone) had coffee and snack with pills.

An okay day. Twitching over left eye, like I used to get, possibly due to drop in Prednisone.

Hissing in ear tonight and tired, guess due to last night. 8:30pm going to bed to read.

2/2/2015 Monday

Woke around 6am stayed awake. Out of bed at 7am.

b/p 112/81 pulse 72

feeling heady, brain fog, this morning.

8:30 122/86 pulse 78

Breakfast and pills Diovan and Toprol ½

Very heady as the morning goes on.

11:15a.m Prednisone 7mgs second day

Out all morning, doctor and store.

Not good mentally, got lost in store, unfamiliar feeling (short lasting)

2:30pm took Prednisone 1mgs makes it 8 today

b/p 5pm 133/84 pulse 79

Heady all day, headache. Having tenderness of scalp also, pain in right cheek.

Left twitchy eye brow, as before prednisone.
Tired tonight.
¼ valium, protonix, sleep 10:30pm

2/3/2015 Tuesday
Woke at 3am with pounding in head, right side, b/p not high. Fell back to sleep in an hour.
Woke at 7am. Up.
b/p 109/80 pulse 71
8:30 breakfast b/p still low
9am b/p 115/81 pulse 76
Coffee to raise b/p and took pills at 10am
11:15am Prednisone 8mgs third day back to it, due to headache, cheek pain and scalp tenderness.
Felt okay today. Worked, writing most of day.
Fell asleep on couch 4-5:30pm woke, slight headache.
6:30pm pills Plavix, Verapamil, aspirin.
7pm Sneezing a lot, then coughing, and breath problem, which I have 'not' had. Windows were open today. Throat has congestion along with upper chest.
9:30 Protonix sleep around 10:30pm

2/4/2015 Wednesday
Slept off and on last night. Fully awake at 5am. Up at 7am. b/p 115/80 pulse 72
8:15 breakfast
9:15am. pills Diovan and Toprol ½
11am prednisone 8mgs fourth day back up to 8
Not great this morning, but not bad.

Slight pain in right side again.

Left side of neck tight, shoulder pulled up, like since neck operation. I guess the way I slept.

Headache before eating lunch, low b/p.

Okay until around 4pm. Laying down reading, almost drifting off to sleep, but then noticed I didn't feel right mentally. Brain Fog, not with it feeling. Neck around carotid artery pulsating, (it does this from time to time) don't know if it has to do with the way I'm laying with my head up on a pillow into my neck or part of GCA. Got up and felt worse, Temperature is 97.7.

Ate dinner around 6pm, took pills Plavix, Verapamil, aspirin. Not better after eating. Still headache on top of head. 7:30pm. still not good.

Bed around 9pm, sleep at 10. woke every two hours during the night.

2/5/2015 Thursday
8am 146/69 pulse 72
8:30 124/80 pulse 78
8:45am Breakfast and pills Diovan and Toprol
9:30 lightheaded
11am Prednisone 5th day on 8mgs
Shower. Lightheaded.

12:30pm. Cardiologist. I have asked them 'not' to give me the PA. We accomplished nothing. PA thought maybe stopping Verapamil and taking Toprol at night instead for the VTack. She also mentioned venous insufficiency is reason my legs, ankles and feet swelling. I told her I did not want any operations on my legs, (striping veins). She argued with me, and I argued back.

Accomplished nothing by going to cardiologist today.

Out from 12:30 – 3pm went to store and walked around for exercise. I felt good. Probably because my blood pressure was up from the doctor's office.

Ate early 4:30pm. dinner.

Bed by 7pm to read, sleep around 9:30.

2/6/2015 Friday

Bad night last night. Went to sleep early woke at 2am and stayed awake until around 4am, took ¼ valium, then off and on sleep until 7am.

8am b/p 124/80 pulse 74

8:30 Breakfast then Diovan and Toprol

Feeling tired this morning, but not bad. Hissing in right ear.

10:30 Prednisone 8mgs sixth day

Laid down for a while being little sleep last night. Still couldn't sleep.

11:30am. started cooking soup standing for an hour, notice my right side, front, back is hurting again.

Had soup for lunch, homemade minestrone.

1:30pm feel okay outside of pain in right side.

Out from 2 till 4:30pm feel okay slight dizziness, not bad.

6pm Dinner had the same as lunch, soup.

7pm headache, and cold, why, I have no idea.

To bed early tonight to read then sleep.
9pm prontonix, 10pm sleep.

2/7/2015 Saturday
Slept 10pm till 2:45am good four hours straight. Then awake. Fell asleep till phone woke me at 7am.
8am 110/72 pulse 69
Breakfast no pills
9:30 b/p 108/80 pulse 79
9:45am Took ½ Toprol only because b/p machine showed heart beat off.
10:45 Prednisone 8mgs seventh day
Still haven't taken Diovan b/p pill still low b/p 117/76 pulse 72. I have a slight headache (forehead) also nasal drip.
12:20pm 128/82 pulse 64, taking Diovan b/p pill.
An okay day, b/p low most of day.
Fell asleep around 4:30pm reading a book on the couch.
6:30 plavix and aspirin with dinner.
7:30pm Verapamil with Ensure. (will have to stay up later tonight to take protonix so it doesn't block the verapamil.
Slight mental problem tonight I notice. Not confused or disoriented, but not right. Kind of anxious nervous.
Bed around 9:30pm to read, lights out 11pm
Slept well, up only three times versus every hour or two.

2/8/2015 Sunday
Woke around 6am. Felt rested.
8am b/p 118/74 pulse 69
8:30breakfast
8:45 Toprol ½
10:15 Prednisone 8mgs eight day
11am b/p 113/74 pulse 72 (still too low to take Diovan) but feeling heady. I don't know how to get pills in order to take every morning with b/p being so low lately, and prednisone.
12pm Diovan 124/78 pulse 74 (very late)
Cooked standing for lunch, right side hurt is back.
An okay day, except for low b/p slight headache.
4:30pm. fell asleep in bed reading, felt better after.
6:30 Plavix with dinner.
7:30pm Verapamil with cookies and Ensure. (headache back).
Seems all I do is lay in bed or sit in a chair, eat and sleep, and still feel lousy. I think it's blood pressure pills, or Prednisone.
Bed by 10pm lights out 11pm

2/9/ 2015 Monday
Woke around 2am then 6am to stay, fairly good sleep.
7:30am 133/82 pulse 79
b/p pills Diovan and Toprol
10:13 Prednisone 8mgs. Ninth day.

Slight headache this morning, nasal drip, slight wheeze.

Cleaning girl here, using cleaning fluids, also windows are open. I started wheezing after 2 ½ hours into cleaning and windows open. Bad wheezing as before I got the Flu. Also short of breath.

Went to lunch burger, fries, soda, while eating neck hurt then dizzy, vertigo.

On to the store, trouble walking around, dizzy, vertigo. Came home, noticed b/p rising, felt better.

6pm dinner, soup, Plavix, Verapamil, aspirin.

Breathing has been okay since I came home from store. I left air-conditioner on and windows open while gone two hours. When home closed windows and had only air on. Seemed better breathing in and no wheezing.

Bed around 9pm, sleep 10pm

2/10/2015 Tuesday

Slept well, woke three times but didn't stay awake.

Up around 6:30am

Wheezing right away this morning. Possible acid reflux, I notice I'm hiccupping a lot after a meal.

7am b/p 120/80 pulse 69

8 breakfast, after b/p pills Diovan and Toprol ½

10:30am Prednisone 8mgs tenth day

Out for blood work per general practitioner's office

Heady around 12 noon,

1:30pm b/p 119/80 pulse 74

Ate lunch at 2pm. homemade soup.

Pretzels 2:45pm

4:30pm laid down a while and read, feeling very hungry (which I never do). Wheezing.

6pm 124/78 pulse 69 (new b/p machine today)

6:15pm dinner, Plavix, Verapamil, aspirin.

Sharp pain behind left breast, down into stomach, or the other way around.

Tired tonight. Protonix 9pm, sleep 10pm

2/11/2015 Wednesday

Slept well last night (crazy dreams, since being on prednisone), woke two times only then fell back to sleep.

Slight headache, woozy not really dizzy.

8am b/p 115/76 pulse 70

Breakfast

Toprol and Diovan around 8:30am

Slight headache

10:45am Prednisone 8mgs. Eleventh day

b/p 116/75 pulse 72

Light headed and wobbly, off balance.

12:15pm very dizzy standing and slight forehead headache.

Not good most of day, dizzy, lightheaded.

b/p 137/82 pulse 72

6pm dinner, pills, Verapamil, Plavix, aspirin, right after burping up fluid (reflux happens a lot lately) also pain under left breast, as last night, but not as bad.

Looked at blood work from yesterday. SED rate up, 48 two weeks ago now 52. Highest in almost a year, inflammation is up. Even on prednisone. See if any doctor calls telling me there's a problem.

Bed by 9pm protonix, asleep by 10:30pm

Woke with a start around 11:30pm. high blood pressure and pulse 155/88 pulse 91.

¼ valium back to sleep.

2/12/2015 Thursday

Woke around 6a.m., throat very raw (from regurgitating yesterday) raspy throat.

8a.m. b/p 118/80 pulse 68

Slightly dizzy this morning when standing.

9am Toprol and Diovan

10:45am. Prednisone 8mgs twelfth day with yogurt and ½ banana and honey.

Not bad, the dizziness gone. Breathing okay.

Air-conditioner fixed today. Worker put something in to take away mold in air handler.

6pm dinner peanut butter sandwich and Ensure with pills, Verapamil, Plavix, aspirin.

Feeling okay, just tired from waking up last night.

Bed 9pm protonix, sleep 9:30pm

2/13/2015 Friday

Woke around 7am

8am b/p 126/80 pulse 72

Feeling okay except for wheezing and congestion in throat.

8:15am. breakfast and pills Diovan and Toprol ½ always a half, unless heart irregular.

Right side hurts early this morning and constipated, little peas or balls again, with white on them.

10:30am Prednisone 8mgs thirteenth day

Feeling okay out from 11am till 1pm

Lunch 1:30pm broccoli, penna, sausage, 3 days in a row.

Right side hurting.

Dinner ½ pork chop, peaches, Ensure, 2 cookies. And pills Verapamil, Plavix, aspirin, all within half hour.

Felt okay today, other than right side hurting.

Feeling slightly nervous tonight around 7pm

Will go to bed early and read.

I fell asleep around 4:30pm. for a few minutes.

Noticed when I got up from computer at 8:30pm I had swooshing sound and heart beat in right ear, this has happened recently I notice. Something new.

b/p 140/82 pulse 72

9pm going to bed, read, then sleep around 10pm

2/14/2015 Saturday

Woke around 6:30am, good night's sleep, woke once around 3am.

8am b/p 113/86 pulse 74

Breakfast oatmeal ½ banana

Diovan and Toprol ½

Not good this morning, slight dizziness and headache. Wheezing.

10:30am. Prednisone 8mgs fourteenth day.

Very heady, laid down around 11am. not good, very cold and woozy.

1pm Lunch salad and peanut butter crackers, chocolate candy.

Not good mentally this morning around lunch time.

Not a good day, headache on top of head and forehead, also not good mentally.

Scared at night and very nervous.

Hardly any sleep. Awake most of night. Sleep then wake, sweats then cold. Took ½ valium, still didn't sleep well.

2/15/2015 Sunday

Up around 8a.m nervous feeling inside. Wheezing.

b/p 121/80 pulse 74

breakfast then Diovan and Toprol ½

10:30 Prednisone 8mgs 15th day on 8mgs

Felt okay today not dizzy.

Swooshing sound in right ear when getting up from sitting.

Cold and hot at times, mostly cold.

Bed around 9pm had cereal at 10:30pm then sleep. Slept from 11pm to 5am, best sleep in a long time. No valium.

2/16/2015 Monday

Awake 5am. but fell back to sleep till 7.

Feel rested. No sweats or chills. Hissing in ears. Wheezing.

8am b/p129/78 pulse 72

Breakfast and Diovan and Toprol ½

10:45am Prednisone 8mgs sixteenth day

Lunch around 1:20pm chicken, egg, fruit and ice cream.

Feeling okay today

Started getting slight headache around 2pm. Funny, after eating. (shouldn't be)

Feeling cold again today, but not cold outside. Temp in the house 77 degrees.

Swooshing sound in right ear again when getting up from sitting position. Then it goes away.

4pm just had homemade smoothie (blue berries, cherries, coconut water, and walnuts.) have a headache anyway so I figure what can the walnuts do if I already have the headache.

Around 7pm headache in middle of eyes, right above nose. Just like months ago.

8:30pm Right ear hissing. Getting hot instead of cold. Had a lot of protein today.

Going to bed soon to read.10pm sleep.

Woke around 2am. fast heart beat and heart beat pounding in head. Ears pounding. Heart skipping beats, and b/p up 150/89 on wrist cuff. Took ¼ valium and some Ensure, stayed awake for an hour trying to calm down. Vtak or sugar low. Had a lot of protein today.

2/17/2015 Tuesday
Woke tired, bad night last night, fast heartbeat and skips.
9am b/p 114/78 pulse 69
9:30am Breakfast then took Diovan and Toprol ½
11am Prednisone 8mgs seventeenth day
12pm out till 3pm have heady feeling, aching in bones over eye brows. Like before prednisone and thought it was sinus infection, turned out Temporal Arteritis or GCA Giant Cell Arteritis.
Home, feel tired, I guess from last night's heart pounding and lack of sleep.
Forehead headache most of day.
6-6:30pm Plavix, Verapamil, aspirin
b/p 132/82 pulse 69
No swooshing sound in right ear after getting up from chair where I've been sitting for almost two hours.
Bed by 9pm reading, Protonix 9:30pm
Sleep around 10. Woke at 1:30am wheezing more than usual.

2/18/2015 Wednesday
Woke around 7am
8am b/p 132/86 pulse 72
Breakfast then Diovan and Toprol ½

Slight headache forehead and nasal drip.

10am feeling okay mentally, almost good, being I'm doing some writing.

11:15am prednisone 8mgs eighteenth day

Out from 12 noon to 2pm. Not feeling well while walking in store. Feel skipped heart beats, and dizzy or lightheaded.

When home still not good, but have an even pulse (heart beat)

b/p 115/75 pulse 68

Feet, ankles and legs swollen this morning and afternoon, into evening. Feeling like worms crawling on bottom of feet, mainly heal on left foot.

Just not feeling well today, brain wise also.

5:30 to 6pm pills, Plavix, Verapamil, aspirin within half hour.

7pm hissing in right ear.

Just read a news article on Chicken Pox and Giant Cell Arteritis. If you've had Chicken Pox you may get Giant Cell Arteritis. (I had Chicken Pox as a child. Mom had shingles when she was in her 70's) Article says you should be on steroid (prednisone) and an antiviral medication. I will ask Rheumy when I see him next week.

Right ear still hissing.

9:30 protonix, 10:30pm small bowl of cheerios.

Slept well, woke once.

2/19/2015 Thursday

Woke this morning grinding teeth, nervous, out of it mentally not thinking correctly, lots of thoughts at one time.

7am up still not good.

7:30 b/p 129/80 pulse 69

Breakfast oatmeal, ½ banana, 4 grapes, raisins, 20 oz. of water and coconut water.

8:15am Diovan and Toprol ½

Not good thinking wise, still nervous feeling.

Bathroom bowel movement very loose, not little hard peas or balls as usual. Two times this morning.

11am Prednisone 8mgs, nineteenth day

Cup of decaf coffee and date nut bread and cream cheese. Feeling cold.

Tried getting my mind on a movie but concentrating is too much, mentally not good.

1pm lunch, meat and veggies, cookie, ice cream

Not good afternoon either.

Took Tylenol around 4pm and laid down, didn't fall asleep. Felt slightly better after resting.

Dinner 6:15pm Verapamil, Plavix, aspirin within the half hour.

8pm slight headache back, also burning in nostril's today, mostly right nostril.

Cold tonight outside in the 30's, freeze warning in effect, and this is South Florida.

9pm protonix then bed to read, 10pm sleep.

Woke with a start around 1:30am pulse 110

b/p 150/99 with wrist cuff so higher with arm cuff. Sweats, pounding in right ear. ¼ valium and tried to relaxation breathing. Minutes later b/p 130/78 pulse 80

Fell asleep, woke 5:30am then awake off and on.

2/20/2015 Friday
Woke tired after last night waking at 1:30am heartbeat, pounding in ear and sweats.

8:15am b/p 119/81 pulse 69

Breakfast cheerios and half banana

Diovan and Toprol ½

Feel okay, not lightheaded or dizzy at 10am.

11a.m. Prednisone 7mgs first day (dropped one milligram, see how I feel, been too nervous, especially last night palpitations)

2pm lunch meat, veggies, ice cream

4pm still feel okay expect for legs hurting, sitting too much today.

8pm good day today, slightly nervous around dinner time 6:15pm otherwise, not bad today. Even did some writing.

Slight headache tonight.

Going to bed soon, tired from last night's heart beat episode.

9pm bed reading, 10 protonix then sleep. Didn't wake till 4:30am. Fell back to sleep till 7am.

2/21/2015 Saturday
Woke 7am. up around 7:15am. Feeling nervous, racing feeling, pulse meter reads 91. Feel like the attacks I get in the middle of night around 1am. Head

bothering me, especially on right eyebrow. Scalp tender feeling. Touch and feel pain on top of head.

b/p 124/81 pulse 79

Breakfast, 8:45am. Diovan and Toprol ½

10am b/p 111/78 pulse 68

11am Prednisone 7mgs second day on seven

Slight headache over right eye.

Feeling okay except for head pain on top of head when I press it.

1pm lunch cabbage, ground beef, carrot, casserole.

Not good after lunch, feeling not right mentally.

Lots of nervousness again, off and on, then the feeling of having to urinate, only small amounts.

I used nasal spray, script over a year old, but it opened the right nostril, and got rid of the bad headache.

Before dinner feeling very nervous as this morning, without sweating. Thought it might be lack of food.

6 to 6:30pm during dinner, Plavix, Verapamil, aspirin, all within the half hour.

7:45pm still feeling nervous, and urinating but dribbles.

Scared.

8:30pm took ¼ valium to settle down, very nervous and scared.

Bed to read. Finally settled down. Took protonix at 9:30pm then sleep.

Woke around 3am. pounding in right ear and bathroom. Stayed awake long time it seemed, then drifted off until 6am.

2/22/2015 Sunday
Not a good night last night. Good till 3am then awake.
Not nervous this morning.
8am b/p 132/81 pulse 79
Breakfast oatmeal then Diovan and Toprol ½
Swooshing in right ear after sitting this morning.
11am Prednisone 7mgs third day
Felt okay this morning before prednisone, hour after not good.
12:10pm Dizzy, lightheaded feeling while sitting in chair working on writing.
b/p 115/81 pulse 76
Went to store around 3pm, not bad walking in store, no pounding in ear, tired though.
Around 5pm my legs started jumping, feet moving, feeling antsy, slightly nervous.
6-6:30pm Plavix, Verapamil, aspirin, all with in the half hour.
9:30pm protonix then sleep.
Woke one time middle of night, stayed awake for quite a while.

2/23/2015 Monday
7am. awake
8am. b/p 102/67 pulse 78
8:30 breakfast

9am 140/83 pulse 76 b/p pills Diovan and Toprol ½

Not good this morning, head in fog, brain not thinking well.

11am Prednisone 7mgs fourth day

Laid down around 11:30am., tired and heady.

Slept little. Up around 1pm to cook lunch. Chicken and greens.

3pm ¼ valium (very nervous) head bad, especially forehead.

I'm sure b/p is up, but not going to check it.

5pm finally feeling calmed down a little. Head still bothering me.

6:30- 7pm took b/p pills, Plavix, Verapamil, aspirin all within half hour.

Still not feeling better. Bad day.

Bed 8:30pm to read.

Protonix 9:30 then to sleep

Woke around 11pm fast heart beat 105, out of it mentally, valium ¼ then back to sleep, till 5am

2/24/2015 Tuesday

Woke at 5am then back to sleep till 6:30.

7:30am up.

8am b/p 135/86 pulse 74

Breakfast and Diovan and Toprol ½

Feel okay.

10am Prednisone 7mgs fifth day

Out around 10:30am. to store. Felt good while out, until 1:30pm. getting lunch, feel slightly dizzy. Burger, fries, soda.

Around 2 feeling nervous while out.

3pm home had ice cream.

Not bad all day.

6-6:30pm dinner and b/p pills Verapamil, Plavix, aspirin, all within half hour.

Slight headache after eating, air-conditioner blowing on me with hydrogen peroxide in it?

Will go to bed around 8:30 protonix at 10pm then sleep. Woke 3 times middle of night, pounding in right ear.

2/25/2015 Wednesday

Woke early 5am, awake three times prior, sweats and pounding in right ear.

7:30am out of bed.

8am 117/72 pulse 76

8:30 breakfast

122/81 pulse 72

b/p pills divovan and Toprol

11am Prednisone 7mg sixth day

Not good this morning head wise. Bad thinking.

Swelling in feet this morning, left foot especially.

2pm still feeling not great.

New cardiologist at 3pm, he's closer to condo. See what he says. I didn't like seeing the PA at the other cardiologist and he talked about changing stents to newer stents in my heart.

6-6:30pm dinner and pills, Verapamil, Plavix, aspirin.

7pm feeling sleepy, tired.

Not good all day, dizzy from this morning, lightheaded more, very swollen feet, eyes, belly, all over body. Seem to be peeing more often also.

I liked new cardiologist, he listened and he knew about Giant Cell Arteritis and PMR. Plus he's easy to talk to because he doesn't spend time looking at a computer screen. I have an Ecco next month and he wants me to have a stress test. But I told him, no, not while I'm on Prednisone. He didn't argue and saw it my way.

Bed before 9pm. Fell asleep then woke at 2am. stayed awake. No valium.

2/26/2015 Thursday

Awake most of night. Up at 6:45.

7am b/p 119/74 pulse 72

Breakfast at 7:30am then took b/p pills Diovan and Toprol ½

Rheumatologist raised Prednisone to 9mgs, because headaches, tenderness of scalp, and swooshing sound in right ear. Temporal arteritis (GCA) flare he thinks. Also SED rate up to 52.

Endo doctor next. Asked lots of questions about heart VTack, but also said possible pre-diabetes. She did an ultra sound of the Thyroid. Have 2 nodules, one 8 milligrams large, other very small not to worry about. She said usually don't do anything unless their 10 milligrams, then biopsy. Said to take fish oil for dry flaky skin. Which I have all over legs, arms and head.

I liked her.

11am took Prednisone 8mgs first day, then another 1mg half hour later. Total 9mgs.

Out from 9am till 12:30pm.

Lunch at 1pm, same as last night sausage, pasta, broccoli, oil and garlic.

Tired from no sleep last night. Will take nap or just lay down.

3:30 – 5pm fell asleep. Woke with headache and puffy eyes.

6-6:30pm. dinner and Verapamil, Plavix, aspirin within half hour.

9pm bed, 9:30 protonix, 9:45 sleep.

2/27/2015 Friday

Woke around 2am, bathroom, laid awake awhile then slept. Woke again around 5am, back to sleep. Up at 7:30. Nervous, jittery, grinding teeth.

8am b/p 115/72 pulse 79

Breakfast

b/p 120/78 pulse 72 pills Diovan and Toprol ½

10am still nervous inside and jittery, grinding teeth, not good mentally.

11am Prednisone 9mgs, second day on higher dose

Around 12pm cold. Laid down, tired, fell in and out of sleep.

1pm lunch, same in three days, penna pasta, sausage, broccoli, oil and garlic, two cookies.

Right after lunch feel skipped heart beats and tired again, also heady. Could go to sleep, but I won't.

b/p 124/80 pulse 70

Not good all day. Heady all day.

6:30 – 7pm dinner, homemade chicken soup, cookies, milk. Plavix, Verapamil, aspirin.

10pm protonix, lights out, sleep.

Woke around 3am to bathroom, pounding in right ear.

Slept well.

2/28/2015 Saturday

Awake around 7am, up at 7:30

8am b/p 132/77 pulse 72

Breakfast and pills Diovan and Toprol ½

10am feeling not good head wise b/p 115/72 pulse 69.

10:15am Prednisone 9mgs third day

Coffee date nut bread and cream cheese.

Not good day mentally after lunch spaghetti meat balls, cookies. Around 2pm

Swooshing in ear was better.

6 – 7pm. dinner cottage cheese and peaches, verapamil, Plavix, aspirin.

Back of neck down low hurts today.

10pm protonix then to sleep around 10:30pm

Woke around 2am stayed awake 5am.

3/1/2015 Sunday

Slept little last night.

When up walking feeling not great mentally, nervous.

Thinking off, making mistakes with stove dials, putting on burner that shouldn't be, wanting the timer instead. Confusion.

8am b/p 120/77 pulse 72

Breakfast

9am b/p 115/69 pulse 74 (no b/p meds yet

10am 110/72 pulse 78 (still no b/p meds.

Thinking has gotten better then when I got up.

10:15am b/p meds Diovan and Toprol ½ with Ensure.

11:30am Prednisone 9mgs fourth day with yogurt, ½ banana, peanut butter crackers.

Went to store, and felt okay head wise, thinking and no headache.

3pm still feeling okay. Had spaghetti and meatballs for lunch at 2pm

Headache, left leg feels numb and tingling.

Feeling not good later head wise, nervous and heady.

In bed at 7:30pm. Too nervous to be up, head feels almost spinning. Feet numb, swollen. Feels like I have socks on, but don't.

Read. Took protonix at 10pm stayed awake long time.

3/2/2015 Monday

Woke around 5am, tried laying on my right side (hard to breathe and painful in chest rib cage) turned back onto left side where I always sleep since neck operation and back to sleep. Woke around 6 then back to sleep. Up at 7am.

7:30am b/p 119/84 pulse 72

Breakfast and pills Diovan and Toprol ½

Grinding teeth this morning, feel swollen around eyes.

10:30am Prednisone 9mgs fifth day

Very cold this morning.

12:30pm Lunch again spaghetti and meatballs and two cookies and milk. Still cold.

Appointment with neurologist today 3:30pm

Going to tell her I think I have start of vascular dementia, at least that's what it feels like when I have 'no' brain. Disoriented at times, confused to time and place. Or possible diabetes beginning, lack of feeling on bottoms of feet feel like I'm wearing socks, when I'm not.

Also swooshing sound in right ear, along with pounding sound.

6pm home from neurologist. Told her of my concerns, brain fog and confusion at times. She really didn't say anything, no testing, wants to see me in six months. She did agree prednisone can make one feel not right in the head.

My right vertebral artery is the one that's not right. Maybe this is why I have so many problems in that ear, like swooshing, and noises that I hear.

b/p in the office was 150/88 pulse 70.

6:30 to 7pm dinner and pills, Verapamil first, Plavix, aspirin, within twenty minutes.

Not good today after lunch at 1pm

Tired tonight, eyes blurry.

Hope to go to bed by nine maybe before.

Right ear popping when swallowing, nasal drip most of day.

Bed around 8:30pm protonix at 9:30 lay awake until around 10pm

Slept then woke at 3:30am stayed awake then slept.

3/3/2015 Tuesday

Up at 7:30.

114/72 pulse 76

8:30am Breakfast and b/p 125/77 pulse 72

Diovan and Toprol ½

Feel okay except for nasal drip and right ear popping as last night.

Eyes swollen.

10:15am Prednisone 9mgs sixth day

12pm bad morning head wise, like yesterday, can't recall words I want to say, and feeling heady.

Hate this feeling having 'no' brain.

6:30pm to 7pm dinner, Plavix, verapamil, aspirin. All within the half hour.

All day out of it brain wise, or head wise. Is it Sugar? Prednisone? Dementia? Which one or how many?

Bed 9pm.10pm Prontonix then sleep.

Woke at 2:30am stayed awake a while then sleep, then woke around 5am.

3/4/2015 Wednesday
7:30 up feel okay.
8am b/p 119/78 pulse 72
Breakfast oatmeal
b/p pills 8:45am Diovan and Toprol
9:30am feel okay outside of nasal drip, head wise okay so far.
10:30am Prednisone 9mgs seventh day
1pm feeling confusion thinking about two doctors getting them mixed up. Confusion while driving.
1:30pm. lunch chicken salad ½ sandwich, fruit, and yogurt. Better thinking after eating lunch.
Out until 3pm feeling a little tired. Lay down around 3:30pm read.
6 – 6:30pm dinner spaghetti and chicken, 2 cookies and milk with pills, Plavix, verapamil, aspirin all within half hour.
In bed by 9pm, protonix at 9:30pm nervous, grinding teeth.
Fell asleep then woke at 3:30am pounding in head, low b/p, stayed awake until 5am. Fell back to sleep for maybe an hour.
Bad night.

3/5/2015 Thursday
Happy Birthday Rose (73 years old today)

Didn't sleep well last night, nervous, grinding teeth.

8:30am 116/79 pulse 68

Breakfast

9:15 pills, Diovan and Toprol ½

Tired this morning. No bowel movement two days. Took teaspoon of olive oil (burns mouth and throat)

11am Prednisone 9mgs eighth day

11am b/p 102/77 pulse 68

12pm. Almost a normal bowel movement. I wonder if the olive oil helped.

Tired this morning.

Felt okay today, inside mouth on cheek sides and tongue, have sores. Feels like tongue is swollen.

1pm out to lunch, Burger King then to store felt okay. Burger king and salt? I don't use salt in meals I cook because of high blood pressure at times and swelling in feet and ankles.

Ice cream around 3pm

Laid down awhile and read.

6 to 6:30pm dinner spaghetti and chicken, two cookies and milk along with meds, Plavix, Verapamil, aspirin.

Bed by 9pm, Protonix at 9:30, sleep by 10:30pm

3/6/2015 Friday

7am woke feeling good. Slept well, woke one time around 2:30am. Restful sleep.

8am b/p128/82 pulse 72

Breakfast then b/p pills Diovan and Toprol ½

11am Prednisone 9mgs ninth day with Ensure drink.

Wheezing this morning, and hard breathing when walking, outside.

12:30pm. back home. Used inhaler, haven't used this in months. Feel better.

Lunch Steak with mushrooms, pears, ice cream and walnuts.

Dinner had rest of steak and mushrooms and ½ banana.

Started to feel nervous, jittery. By bed time I was totally off the wall.

Bed around 9 took ¼ valium for nervousness and heady feeling. Took protonix at 9:30 and fell asleep.

Woke around 2am, fell asleep, then woke at 5am stayed awake.

3/7/2015 Saturday

Woke early and read awhile, then fell asleep for few minutes. Out of bed at 7:45am

8:30 b/p 120/81 pulse 71

Breakfast oatmeal then pills Diovan and Toprol ½

11am Prednisone 9mgs tenth day

1:30pm lunch sausage, penna, broccoli, olive oil, garlic and onion. Ice cream cake old friend came for surprise visit.

3pm started to feel heady.

4pm still not good, had two pretzel sticks.

6-6:30pm dinner, same as lunch, two cookies and milk with pills, Plavix, verapamil, aspirin.

Going to bed 8:30pm, Protonix 9:30pm

Slept well except for feeling cold when awake. Woke 2 times, woke 5am with nightmare, nervous inside body, eyes swollen.

3/8/2015 Sunday

Up at 6:30, changed clocks last night hour back.

8am b/p 117/72 pulse 74

Breakfast

9:15am b/p 114/75 pulse 69 (no b/p pills yet)

10:15am Still low b/p but took pills. Diovan and Toprol ½

11:30 Prednisone 9mgs eleventh day

Around 12:30pm. not good, head wise. Hour after prednisone.

1:30pm lunch, chicken, potato, greens, ice cream.

Went to store (okay in store) home around 3:30pm

Around 4pm started getting cramps in my left foot toes. (bad, like when I was on higher dose prednisone)

6-6:30pm took meds, Plavix, verapamil, aspirin. With dinner salad with chicken, cookies and milk.

7pm still having cramps/spasms seems to be on the left side of my body, into my chest and left arm.

Took ¼ valium to try and relax muscles in body, get rid of the spasms. b/p 130/82 pulse 80

8:15pm calming down a little, relaxing muscles, valium working, I guess. Might need to take more before bed. Don't want spasms waking me up tonight. Also scared.

9pm ¼ valium, then protonix 9:30pm. Slept off and on, mostly awake, all night.

3/9/2015 Monday
Bad night last night, awake a lot, tight muscles.
8:30am. b/p 125/78 pulse 80, skipped beats.
Breakfast with pills Diovan and Toprol ½
Tired this morning, very tired.

Bad day yesterday afternoon and evening, felt like I was having a stroke with the muscles spasms I had. From facial check, left side, breast and arm, left side, foot, toes, left side. (maybe took prednisone too soon after b/p pills)

I've noticed this morning I'm getting slight pains/aches in the right side of sinus, in cheek and above right eyebrow also into side of head in front of right ear.

11am Prednisone 8mgs down 1mg first day, hoping this stops the muscle spasms.

12pm muscle spasms, hurting into bone under arm pit.

1pm lunch squash, mushrooms sautéed and ½ Ensure drink.

Laid down most of day hoping muscles will feel better. Don't like any of these feelings.

5pm sitting in chair writing this.

6-6:30pm dinner, Plavix, Verapamil, aspirin.

7:20pm Feel better with spasms, not hurting underneath arm pits on bone anymore. Possibly the prednisone too close to the blood pressure meds yesterday, or the drop to 8mgs today from 9mgs yesterday.

9:20pm Protonix then sleep.

Slept very well, woke one time, no spasms.

3/10/2015 Tuesday

Woke 7am and felt well.

8am b/p 126/81 pulse 66

8:30am Breakfast and pills Diovan and Toprol ½

11am Prednisone 8mgs second day

Feeling okay this morning.

1pm Swooshing in right ear after getting up from sitting.

1:30pm lunch, pork chop, with veggies, ice cream

3:30pm still feel okay, other than right ear crunching when swallowing. Even took shower this morning being I didn't feel bad. Hard to shower. I've lost my balance.

4pm slight headache.

6-6:30pm dinner cereal and pills Plavix, Verapamil and aspirin.

Eyes feel swollen and belly swollen today.

9pm bed, protonix 9:30pm ½ valium then sleep.

Slept well, up two times.

3/11/2015 Wednesday

Woke around 7am after vivid dreams. Not a nightmare, but just very vivid, as I've been having all along being on prednisone.

Midway down legs they are numb, feet included. Like cut off at the calf.

Got up and walked to the bathroom, they came back to life. But I felt very nervous, shaky, jittery.

Felt pulse was high. I tried to lie back in bed, but couldn't, too nervous, and feeling I had to move bowels. I thought low sugar and took sugar test 107 (not low). Usually reads around 85.

7:30am b/p 148/76 pulse 94. High b/p, usually low in morning, low so I have to wait to take pills. I was told not to take blood pressure meds unless it's 120.

In kitchen I drank some milk. I had only cereal for dinner last night so maybe electrolytes off.

Had coconut water, with boiled egg and half banana.

7:40am Took b/p pills Diovan and Toprol ½

Laid down for a while to get jittery a feeling I'm out of my body, also moved bowels. I notice when I get this jittery feeling I have to go to move bowels.

10am b/p 137/81 pulse 72 (feeling better) but still not great. I also wonder if it's the drop in Prednisone. I know it plays havoc with your blood sugar.

11am Prednisone 8mg third day

Feeling awful this morning, nervous, jittery, and having to go to the bathroom.

1:30pm. lunch chicken, spaghetti and mushrooms, ice cream for dessert.

2:15 feeling better. Maybe just needed food.

Good afternoon. Felt much better.

6-6:30pm dinner, same as lunch, chicken, spaghetti, mushrooms, piece of chocolate. Pills, Plavix, verapamil, aspirin.

8pm feeling okay, just tired. Bed early tonight.

9:20pm Protonix, asleep by 10:30pm

Woke around 2am with chills, then sweats. Stayed awake for maybe an hour, then fell back to sleep. Woke around 5am then back to sleep till 8am.

3/12/2015 Thursday

Woke out of a sound sleep dreaming. Cold, then hot.

Took temperature 97.6 when cold then minutes later sweats 98.7. Interesting.

8am b/p 125/74 pulse 72

Breakfast then pills Diovan and Toprol ½

Feeling mentally off and light headed.

Ultra sound at new cardiologist, didn't see doctor, just test.

11am Prednisone 8mgs fourth day taken with Ensure.

Still not good mentally, lightheaded walking in store.

12:30pm home b/p 118/76 pulse 80

Lunch. Same as the day before, spaghetti, chicken, mushrooms, cookies and milk.

2pm after lunch feeling okay.

Okay all afternoon, even no swooshing in right ear, or pounding.

b/p 126/81 pulse 76

6:30-7pm dinner baked potato with broccoli on top. Pills Plavix, verapamil, aspirin all within the half hour.

Still feeling okay. Except for back, right side hurting after going to store this morning.

No bowel movement today.

9:30pm protonix sleep at 10pm

Phone woke me at 11:30pm, totally confused, disoriented, scared, heart pounding. Wrong number.

Took ¼ valium and stayed awake for half an hour, then slept till 2:30am, fell back to sleep till 4:45 then awake at 6 and stayed awake. Sweats mostly, still some chills.

3/13/2015 Friday

Bad night last night.

8:30am sugar 95, b/p 141/83 pulse 72

Breakfast then pills Diovan and Toprol ½

Had bowel movement, still small hard pieces for almost a year.

11am b/p 124/81 pulse 70

Sugar 99. Seems low after breakfast at 8:30am

Feeling out of it mentally, not thinking good at all. Got up this morning and worked on my writing, now I'm out of it mentally. (What the heck is this? Alzheimer's? Vascular Dementia? What?)

11:10am Prednisone 8mgs fifth day.

12:48pm still not good mentally. Lunch around 1pm chicken burger.

Not good today, out of it mentally all day.

6:30 – 7pm dinner, and pills Plavix, verapamil, aspirin.

Still not good. Almost feel I have infection somewhere, but where?

Tired today, little sleep last night, hope to go to sleep early.

8:30pm. bed to read. 9pm protonix, then sleep. Woke around 1:30am pounding and sweating, b/p okay.

Slept well.

3/14/15 Saturday

Woke around 7am, felt okay.

8:30 b/p 127/84 pulse 69

Breakfast and pills Diovan and Toprol ½

Bowel movement tiny hard peas as usual.

11am b/p 140/80 pulse 72

11am Prednisone 8mgs sixth day, had egg and muffin with pill.

Took suppository and went to bathroom almost normal.

Not feeling bad.

Pretty good day today. Some spasms under left breast in rib cage, but not bad.

I did notice b/p was in the 140's. I do feel better when b/p is higher than 110's and lower.

Bed 9:30, protonix 10pm sleep at 10:30pm

3/15/2015 Sunday
8am b/p 126/83 pulse 69
Breakfast then pills at 8:30 Diovan and Toprol ½
Aching this morning. Woke aching, in upper legs on sides shoulders, neck, muscles, can't relax them even when lying down.
11am Prednisone 8mgs seventh day.
12pm not good mentally. Slightly out of it.
In pain most of the day.
Hard trying to relax when my body won't let me.
5:45 – 6:15 dinner and pills, Plavix, verapamil, aspirin.
Feeling better, don't know why. Pain finally left body like - blink of an eye.
Left leg and foot has been swollen all day.
Bed around 9pm protonix at 9:30pm. sleep by 10pm
Woke 12:30am., then again at 2am, then 4am, stayed awake until 6am. then fell asleep.

3/16/2015 Monday
8am b/p 110/81 pulse 79
8:30 breakfast no pills
9:30am 125/80 pulse 89 took pills Diovan & Toprol ½
Body in pain and feels tired this morning.
11:15am Prednisone 7mgs first day down from eight after seven days.
An okay day. A lot of work writing and editing. So I guess I had a mind about me.

5:45pm to 6:15pm dinner and pills, Plavix, verapamil, aspirin.

Slight headache tonight at 7pm.

Hope to go to bed early, tired, little sleep this morning. Bed 9pm, protonix 9:30pm then sleep 10pm.

Vivid dreams. Woke a few times.

3/17/2015 Tuesday

Woke early 5am, back to sleep till 7:30am

8am 112/90 pulse 79

8:30 breakfast still low b/p

9:30am took pills, Diovan and Toprol ½

Lower belly cramps this morning, like going to get diarrhea, but have small hard peas instead.

Swooshing in right ear after sitting.

11am Prednisone 7mgs second day

Still feeling cramping inside lower intestines, left overs last night, broccoli, chicken?

Not good mentally when going out.

12:30pm out for lunch burger, fries and dr. pepper.

Even in store not good mentally, breathing is off, wheezing slightly.

Home by 2:30pm., still not great.

6 to 6:30pm dinner, steak and greens, cookies and milk. b/p Pills Plavix, verapamil, aspirin all in half hour.

Eyes very blurred later in afternoon, and feel swollen. Did a lot of work with eyes today, reading and writing.

Hope for bed early tonight.

I'd love to know why I yawn so much. Before meals, after meals, morning and evening, like now at 8:10pm I yawn and my nose runs - Interesting.

b/p 121/71 pulse 66

Slight wheezing from regurgitation.

9:30pm protonix, sleep by 10:30.

Woke around 1:30am couldn't breathe, belly pushing into chest, throat feels raspy (reflux) heart beat slow.

Stayed awake for about ½ hour then back to sleep.

3/18/2015 Wednesday

Woke a number of times this morning since 1:30am. Saw 4am then 6am, fell back to sleep woke 7:45am.

8:30am b/p 129/81 pulse 69

Breakfast, then pills Diovan and Toprol ½

Belly still bloated and feeling into chest. Also still hic cupping (burping) as yesterday.

11:15am. Prednisone 7mgs third day

Still burping up fluid, belly very blown up.

Stomach not good all day. A lot of burping, hic cupping, belly blown up.

1:30pm. Lunch chicken soup.

6:15 – 7pm dinner, baked potato, pumpkin and yogurt, 2 cookies and milk.

Pills different order tonight. Maybe Plavix right away at dinner is bothering stomach. So I took Verapamil, Plavix, aspirin all within half an hour.

Hope to go to bed early, if stomach calms down.
9pm bed to read. 10pm protonix (stomach pill), then sleep.
Slept well, woke twice. Okay no heart beat problems.

3/19/2015 Thursday
Woke around 6am, slightly nervous. Had only ½ baked potato last night for dinner.
8am 126/81 pulse 72
8:30am breakfast and pills, Diovan and Toprol ½
Intestinal pains this morning, then moved bowels, almost normal, still small hard peas with white fuzz.
11am Prednisone 7mgs fourth day
Sneezing and congestion in throat this morning.
Very nervous most of the day.
6-6:30pm dinner, pills Verapamil, Plavix, aspirin, same as last night.
Hope to go to bed early. 9:30pm protonix and sleep
Woke two times then 5:30am. felt no blood in body, not cold or hot.
Fell asleep and dreamed, woke, fell asleep and dreamed. This happened a few times.

3/20/2015 Friday
Woke around 7am. feeling slightly nervous. When up standing, very nervous, grinding teeth.

Took blood sugar 90. Breathing is fine, pulse slightly high. Pulse meter 80's, oxygen 97/96.

8:30 b/p 112/72 pulse 66

Breakfast (no pills yet)

9am b/p 149/78 pulse 70 took pills, Diovan and Toprol ½

Still feeling nervous and ear hissing.

11am Prednisone 7mgs fifth day.

11:15am till 2:30pm out, blood work, lunch then store.

Feeling nervous and out of it mentally all day. Right ear very sensitive to sounds. Hurts my head inside hearing loud sounds.

4:30pm laid down to read for a while, tired, wanted sleep but couldn't. Feel cold, and scared.

6pm before dinner feel chills, nervous and scared.

b/p 147/76 pulse 80

Dinner Oatmeal and Ensure, pills verapamil, Plavix, aspirin.

Slight headache most of afternoon, wondering if it's walnuts I had yesterday.

Bed around 9pm. Protonix 9:45pm. sleep.

3/21/2015 Saturday

Woke around 5am, then finally awake, awake at 6am. Nervous, grinding teeth.

7:30am b/p 106/71 pulse 70 nasal drip

Breakfast at 8am b/p 122/76 pulse b/p pills Diovan and Toprol ½

Still nervous but not as bad.

Moved bowels this morning, cramps, like diarrhea, turned out small soft pieces, not hard peas like usual. I've been eating can pumpkin, is this helping?

10:30am Prednisone 7mgs sixth day took pills with nut cream cheese.

11 - 12noon out to store shopping. Feel okay in store, trying to walk fast up and down isles. Only one lightheadedness episode. No pain or aching. Different than yesterday when body full of pain.

12:30pm lunch, sandwich ham and turkey

3pm Laid down, tired and cold.

Up around 4:30pm slight headache and out of it mentally, Scared feeling, as other day. Possible aura before migraine, from nut cream cheese at 11am. Just a thought. (don't like the out of mind feeling, this is when I feel I'm getting dementia.

5:30 dinner, penna, sausage, broccoli garlic and oil.

Pills, Verapamil, Plavix, aspirin.

Still not good mentally, plus slight forehead headache and runny nose from sneezing.

Bed around 9pm protonix 9:30, sleep by 10pm

3/21/2015 Sunday

5:30am awake, laid in bed till getting out of bed around 7am.

8am b/p 157/88 pulse 79 company coming.
Breakfast and pills Diovan and Toprol ½
10:30am Prednisone 7mgs seven day
Bad all day so far, mentally feeling not there.
Spasms under left breast this morning then again at 3pm. Still not good.
6 – 6:30pm dinner and pills Verapamil, Plavix, aspirin.
Not good all day, out of it mentally, even with company talking. Felt In a fog.
Bed around 8:30pm protonix at 9:30pm and sleep around 10pm.
Woke at 1:30am and stayed awake with sweats. Finally took ¼ valium at 4am and fell asleep until 7am.

3/23/2015 Monday
8am b/p 125/82 pulse 80
Breakfast and pills Diovan and Toprol ½
Tired this morning, probably due to valium at 4am.
10:30am Prednisone 6mgs first day down from 7.
Fairly good today, mentally, not like yesterday. Even did some writing.
Later in day spasms in mid-section.
5:50 – 6pm headache top of head. Dinner, and pills, verapamil, Plavix, aspirin. Bed early tonight.
Bed at 9pm to read, 9:30pm protonix sleep 10pm woke at 11:30pm. wide awake. Took ¼ valium back

to sleep, then woke around 2am, then again around 4. Bad night, hardly any sleep.

3/24/2015 Tuesday
Woke 5:45am stayed awake, out of bed 6:30am. Wheezing.
b/p 117/74 pulse 80 high pulse this morning.
7:30am breakfast oatmeal
b/p 101/77 pulse 79 (no pills, b/p too low.)
8:30am b/p 127/84 pulse 75
Pills Diovan and Toprol ½
Cardiologist this morning 9:15am. (says Echo okay, still wants stress test and again I said, "No. Not till I'm off prednisone." See him in July next visit. b/p in his office was 145/80.
Feeling slightly lightheaded this morning.
Went for walk in store, still light headed at times.
10:30am Prednisone 6mgs second day on six.
After sitting swooshing sound in right ear, didn't have it yesterday at all. Today belly is blow up, yesterday it wasn't.
Not great today, but not bad. Tired mostly, from little sleep last night.
Left leg, ankle and foot swollen, along with belly.
5:30 – 6pm dinner and pills, verapamil, Plavix, aspirin. Slight headache before and after.
Slept fairly well tonight, bed 9pm, prontonix.
Slept and woke around 2am, then 6am.

3/25/2015 Wednesday
Up early, 7am. 8am b/p 122/74 pulse 76
Breakfast and pills, Diovan and Toprol ½
Doctor Rheumy
11:45am Prednisone 6mgs. Third day on 6
Okay until sitting in Burger king, then pain in back and hips.
2pm home from store and doctor, feeling okay today.
Dinner verapamil, Plavix, aspirin.
7pm b/p 145/88 pulse 80.
Hope to go to bed early. 8:30 bed, 9:30 protonix, turned out light 10:30pm ¼ valium. Slept okay.

3/26/2015 Thursday
Woke early 5:30am, on and off back to sleep, out of bed around 7:30am
8am b/p 126/72 pulse 76
Breakfast oatmeal, then Diovan and Toprol ½
Swooshing in ear early this morning, after sitting then standing. I thought it was gone, but I guess not.
Not as nervous this morning as usual. Not grinding teeth.
10:30am Prednisone 6mgs fourth day.
A lot of pain today in my back. Stress from yesterday probably. Stress doesn't go well with this disease PMR/GCA. But how does one get away from stress when their living with it?
1pm lunch sausage, broccoli and pasta, olive oil and garlic, ice cream for dessert.

Tired today, laid down around 3:30 - 5pm, couldn't sleep.

6 – 6:30pm dinner, cheerios and half banana and milk. Pills, verapamil, Plavix, aspirin.

Feeling a little edgy tonight. Not like most of the day, I was relaxed. Just hope I can sleep tonight.

9pm bed to read, 9:30 protonix, 10:30 to sleep.

Woke maybe an hour after I fell asleep, totally out of it. Confused, disoriented. I thought sugar, being I'd only had cheerios for dinner, and drank some Ensure sitting next to bed. I began to feel better.

3/27/2015 Friday

Woke around 3am and slept off and on till 7am then out of bed. Feeling shaky right away, and wheezing.

8am b/p 127/81 pulse 76

Coconut water right away then Breakfast waffle with butter, ½ banana, 5 grapes.

Pills, Diovan and Toprol ½

8:20am. not as nervous now, but still am. I wonder Sugar? When waking up out of bed (shaky)

10:30am Prednisone 6mgs fifth day

Not very good this morning still. Headache, and when I shake my head it hurts on top right sinus area, GCA. Like before prednisone.

1pm lunch, while eating spasms under left breast.

1:30pm after lunch ¼ valium. Hoping to calm down.

Went to store, while in store spasms in left breast or behind and underneath. Seems I'm getting them back again.

6 to 6:30pm dinner (same as lunch) still not good, bad chills as usual when ready to eat, slight headache and spasms left upper body. Hissing in right ear, and nervous, confusion slight. Same at 7:40pm

Even slight headache now. 9pm bed to read, 9:30pm protonix, sleep by 11pm

3/28/2015 Saturday

Woke at 3am, then again at 5 then off and on finally around 6:30 feeling body nervous, comes on slowly and intensifies. I got out of bed, shaky, jittery, grinding teeth. (might be adrenal glands starting to work coming down on prednisone.)

8am b/p 127/81 pulse 72

Breakfast oatmeal

Then b/p pills Diovan and Toprol ½

8:30am Still nervous and jittery.

11am Prednisone 6mgs sixth day

Not good this morning, stomach cramps like diarrhea, had small balls, then very loose stool, almost water. Cramps.

1:30pm. lunch, chicken, mushrooms, carrots, onion, bean salad, two cookies.

Feel bad all day. Belly blown up after bathroom diarrhea.

6-6:30pm dinner, cereal, and pills verapamil, Plavix, aspirin.

9pm bed to read. 9:30 protonix, sleep by 10:30pm

Woke around 12 midnight very nervous, high pulse 95 and confusion.

3/29/2015 Sunday

Woke around 6am and stayed awake, very nervous, high pulse, shaky, grinding teeth. Tired, reading in bed to relax, had coconut water also. Finally up at 7:30am.

8am 134/81 pulse 70

Breakfast oatmeal and pills Diovan and Toprol ½

9:45am not as nervous.

10:30am Prednisone 6mgs seventh day

Feeling like I am sick today, have an infection somewhere in body. Eyes feel swollen and head is just off, foggy. B/p seems to be okay, not high, or low. And not feeling any skipped beats.

Don't know if this is the drop in prednisone or what, it's the 7th day on 6mgs of prednisone.

6 – 6:30pm dinner, waffle with butter, ½ banana, cup of oatmeal, and scrambled egg, water, no milk.

Still not right after eating dinner, feel like illness in body, UTI? I don't know.

Hope to go to bed early tonight. 9pm bed to read, 9:30 protonix, then sleep. Woke around 1am nervous, spasms/cramps in feet and leg, took Ensure and ¼ valium. Back to sleep till 5am, bathroom, then slept till 6:15am.

3/30/2015 Monday
8am 120/78 pulse 80
Breakfast, oatmeal
8:30 pills Diovan and Toprol ½

Swooshing sound in right ear after standing from sitting.

10:30am Prednisone 6mgs eighth day

11am – 2pm out to store and lunch. Burger, fries and dr. pepper.

Right side of mid-section aches, at times, sharp pain as a few months ago when I thought it was a pulled muscle. Don't know what this is, possibly intestinal.

Hurting badly while out, right leg, foot, hip, almost feel as I did before starting prednisone. (a lot of inflammation)

6:30pm – 7pm dinner and pills, verapamil, Plavix, aspirin.

Urinating very little today.

9pm bed to read. 9:30 protonix, then sleep by 10:30pm. Woke around 3am and stayed awake.

3/31/2015 Tuesday
Up around 7am feel okay, little sleep after 3am this morning.
8am 121/69 pulse 72
Breakfast then pills Diovan and Toprol ½

Feel okay this morning head wise, and body wise, except for sneezing and left ear squashing when swallowing.

10:30am Prednisone 6mgs ninth day

Had pumpkin, ½ banana, honey and cinnamon with prednisone.

Belly blown up today, as yesterday, but not hurting as much as yesterday.

1:30 – 3:30pm out to lunch and store shopping. Felt chills before eating, then walking in store lower back hurt and slightly light headed, after eating.

Tired when home. Lay on couch around 5:15pm and read.

6:30pm – 7pm dinner ½ sandwich ham and turkey, and some chicken salad, two cookies and milk, with pills, verapamil, Plavix, aspirin within the half hour.

New sugar meter read 134, 126 after eating.

Bed early tonight, tired, eyes sleepy.

9pm bed to read, 9:30pm protonix, 10:30 sleep.

Slept till 1am, then awake disoriented, drank some Ensure.

Stayed awake even after taking ½ valium all night.

4/1/2015 Wednesday

Up most of the night, terrible night, disoriented first then cramps/spasms, and pain in legs, feet and mid-section.

6am bad Charlie horse in leg and feet.

8am out of bed, can't sleep.

b/p 126/78 pulse 72

Breakfast waffle, egg, ½ banana drank coconut water for cramping. I guess this is a FLARE.

9am Diovan and Toprol ½

11am Prednisone 6mgs tenth day

In a lot of pain today, spasms/cramps, wonder if it's the lunch I had yesterday, pizza bread, gluten?

Have tried drinking coconut water, Gatorade and plain water, but still have aching. Flare, I guess. (very painful). Also feet are purple, and belly big.

All day felt bad, in pain.

Dinner 5:30pm – 6pm verapamil, Plavix, aspirin.

Bed by 9:30pm to read, took protonix. Sleep by 10:30pm. Woke at 2am. took ¼ valium, fell back to sleep. On and off sleep till 6:30am fully awake.

4/2/2015 Thursday

8 am feel blood pressure is high. Wrist cuff reads 140/80.

Breakfast oatmeal and pills Diovan and Toprol ½

Feel slightly off this morning. Feel like beginnings of dementia, and maybe it is.

Hurting again this morning, almost spasms/cramps but not happening.

10:30am Prednisone 6mgs eleventh day

Not great today. Head is off and top of head into sides feel odd. Headache later in day.

Bad around 4:30pm.

Sugar is 124. Not high, not low.

Dizzy surge around 5:30pm, haven't had that in a while, wonder if it's the lower prednisone?

Bad headache on top front of head. Took Tylenol. Hope to sleep early.

4/3/2015 Friday

Slept off and on last night, cramps/spams in leg and back. I may go to 7mgs of prednisone today instead of 6mgs. Maybe it was too soon a drop.

8:30am 118/86 pulse 79

Sugar 80 before eating

Breakfast and pills Diovan and Toprol ½

Tired this morning, was awake every two hours last night.

10:30am two hours after eating breakfast.

Prednisone 7mgs, increase from 6 because the way I've been feeling for a few days, headache and muscle spasms.

12:30pm sugar 102 before lunch. Very hungry stomach, (never have this) hamburger and salad, then ice cream. Hard to breathe for some reason. Slight wheeze.

Felt odd these past days. Out of it mentally, in a fog. Scared at times.

Bad day, lung wise and head wise. Breathing problems, hard to intake air and wheezing a lot.

Tired at night. To bed by 9pm to read, protonix 9:30pm then fell asleep right away at 10pm. Woke at 11pm out of it. Had half Ensure thinking maybe I didn't have enough to eat for dinner.

Woke at 3am, then 6am.

4/4/2015 Saturday
Woke early around 6:30am, out of bed around 7am. b/p 120/76 pulse 79

Breakfast and pills Diovan and Toprol ½

10:45am Prednisone 7mgs up again second day. Still not feeling good, in pain.

2:30pm to 4pm fell asleep, had ice cream and two pieces of chocolate, got really sleepy and fell asleep.

5:30pm to 6:30pm dinner and pills, verapamil, Plavix, aspirin.

Still feeling not good, mentally, head wise, depressed maybe due to living like this. If this is called living?

Hope to go to bed early, still tired at 7pm.

Bed at 9pm to read, 9:30pm protonix, 10:15pm turned light out. Slept till 1am, awake, slept till 3am, slept till 4:45am, stayed awake for an hour, then fell asleep till 8am. Not a very bad night.

4/5/2015 Sunday
8am b/p 118/78 pulse 76

Breakfast oatmeal, piece of bacon.

8:30am pills, Diovan and Toprol ½.

10:45am Prednisone 6 and ½ this is the first day taking half.

Worked on writing today.

5:45pm to 6:30pm egg sandwich and peaches, pills Verapamil, Plavix, aspirin.

Eyes very sleepy today. Guess because I woke at 5am.

9pm bed, 9:30pm protonix, 10pm sleep. Woke out of sound sleep around 11:30pm. with fast heart beat and high blood pressure 179/91 pulse 106. Took ¼ valium, it was down twenty minutes later, and back to sleep.

4/6/2015 Monday

Woke 6am, stayed in bed, slept off and on, out of bed 7:15am. Feel okay. Eyes sleepy, swollen maybe.

8am b/p 126/78 pulse 79

Breakfast cheerios with cinnamon and pills Diovan an Toprol ½

Feeling not bad, have my brain to write at least.

11:20am Prednisone 6 and ½ second day on this.

Still feeling okay mentally. (I wonder if it has to do with my blood pressure going up last night, along with my heart rate. Blood getting to my brain) just a thought.

An okay day, got a lot done writing, mind thinking well, almost normal.

3:30pm got real sleepy reading and fell asleep for half an hour.

6:30pm to 7pm dinner, same as lunch, spaghetti and chicken, two cookies and grapes.

Forehead and above headache after eating. 7:45pm sugar is 135 a little high, cookies and grapes I guess.

Eyes swollen, belly swollen and tired again.
9pm bed to read, 9:45 protonix, 10:30 sleep.
Slept well.

4/7/2015 Tuesday
Woke around 7am slept well last night, woke once at 3:30am, then back to sleep.
Sweats after waking, took sugar 75, lowest it's been.
8am. b/p 128/83 pulse 71
Breakfast oatmeal, raisins, cinnamon. Coconut water to drink.
Pills Diovan and Toprol ½
11am Prednisone 6 and ½ third day. Think I feel better adding the half but not sure.
1pm burger king fries, and dr. pepper, always feel better when I have this. WHY? Is it the salt?
After lunch walked around store at a good pace. Not in pain or out of breath.
6:15pm to 7pm dinner, squash, mushrooms, and spaghetti from yesterday. Pills, verapamil, Plavix, aspirin.
Belly blown up before eating dinner, and after, still at 8:15pm
Going to bed to read 9pm, 10pm protonix. Sleep by 11pm

4/8/2015 Wednesday
Woke at 4am. deep dream, then sweats and fast heartbeat. b/p 150/90 pulse 88 with wrist cuff. Sugar

77. Had coconut water, then a little Ensure 4:30am sugar 79. But stayed awake after that.

Out of bed around 7:30am. Sugar 78.

8:30am b/p 139/78 pulse 71

Breakfast oatmeal, ½ banana, some grapes, coconut water and tap water.

Tired and achy this morning, from being up a while, I guess.

11am 6 and ½ Prednisone fourth day

Very tired this morning and into the afternoon, also wheezing a lot.

2pm. Lunch ½ egg sandwich, ½ banana, ice cream.

3pm cooking, lower back hurts. Bones hurt after trying to sleep on my right side this morning, also wheezing started.

5:30pm sugar 135 (high)

6pm – 6:30pm dinner, stew. Pills verapamil, Plavix, aspirin.

Still tired, sleepy eyes (swollen all day)

Hopefully will sleep tonight more than five hours.

Slept well all night, up one time around 2am, then woke at 4:45am wide awake, and started sweating, sugar 76. b/p normal.

4/9/2015 Thursday

Woke 5:45am and stayed up sugar 76.

7:15 b/p 135/81 pulse 78

Breakfast and pills Diovan and Toprol ½

Okay this morning, a little out of it thinking wise, not remembering flowers names that I should know.

Foot doctor this morning, asked if I was taking medication for diabetes. "No." I said. "I haven't been diagnosed with diabetes."

He seems to think I do have hypoglycemia precursor to diabetes.

Had a slight panic attack while waiting in his office. Toe nails clipped. I can't do them anymore because of big belly I have.

11:30 sugar 87, going to take Prednisone 6 and ½, fifth day. Decaf coffee, piece of bacon, ¼ cup of left over oatmeal from this morning.

Still nervous.

Lunch, stew, ice cream for dessert.

Slight pain over right side of head has lasted all day, it is now 5:30pm. getting ready to eat dinner.

Tired and headache pain most of day.

5:30 - 6pm dinner stewed chicken, cookies and milk.

8:30pm bed to read, slight headache all day, still now. Protonix 9:30, sleep 10:15pm

4/10/2015 Friday

Woke around 6am, sweats and nervous, sugar 78. Had small glass of coconut water and laid down. b/p normal by wrist cuff, 128/76. Half hour later sugar is 90. Moved bowels right away this morning.

8:20am b/p 135/85 pulse 79, skipped heart beats. Breakfast oatmeal. Diovan and Toprol ½ hissing in right ear and feel tired.

11:30am Prednisone 6 and ½ sixth day.

1:30pm lunch, chicken, macaroni and cheese, cole slaw, ice cream.

4pm laid down on couch, tired, read and fell asleep off and on. 5:30pm lying there, hissing in right ear, I notice I was not thinking right, mentally, scared. Got up and took sugar 120 which was fine.

b/p high 142/86 pulse 79 I did have pretzels and chicken salad from store, salt.

6:15pm – 6:45pm dinner and pills, verapamil, Plavix, aspirin. Still not feeling right mentally, hissing in right ear, and shaky.

7:45pm still not good, but feeling tired.

9pm bed, 9:30 protonix, 10:30 sleep. Woke around 2am, started sweating, took sugar 90, then some coconut water, sweats stopped.

4/11/2015 Saturday

Woke at 2am, then 4am, then 6am and stayed awake.

8am b/p 121/82 pulse 73

Breakfast oatmeal ½ banana, and grapes. Feeling a little light headed this morning.

8:30am pills Diovan and Toprol ½

Still light headed.

11am Prednisone 6 and ½ seventh day

Not great this morning.

1:30pm lunch, steak, potato, string beans, ice cream. Have bad chills up right side of back while eating. This has happened now for a few months. Feeling to pee a lot also today. UTI?

3:30pm still have chills.

Had nuts and peanut butter crackers around 4pm. I usually get a headache, but I'm watching the Masters golf tournament, and want to celebrate my old days playing golf.

6-6:30pm not great mentally, brain fog. Took pills with dinner, verapamil, Plavix, aspirin. With cheerios and ½ banana. Eyes feel swollen, and forehead headache. Still not good mentally, almost depressed.

9pm bed to read, 10pm Protonix, 10:30pm sleep.

Woke around three times.

4/12/2015 Sunday

Woke around 6am then sweats, took sugar 95, didn't take anything, no coconut water.

8am out of bed, tired this morning, and aching, upper legs, mainly.

8:30am 125/75 pulse 72

Breakfast oatmeal then pills Diovan and Toprol

Feeling tired this morning still at 10:30.

11am Prednisone 6 and ½ eighth day.

Feeling down again wanting to cry, today as yesterday.

3:45pm still feeling down. Watching the Masters on TV. Possibly old memories bringing me down.

Swollen left ankle today as yesterday. Laid down and put leg up watching TV.

6:30 – 7pm cheerios and pills Verapamil, Plavix, aspirin.

Nervous most of day after lunch, maybe coffee or prednisone?

Scared tonight, most of day.
9pm bed to read, 9:45pm protonix, 10:30 sleep.
Slept fairly well, woke 3times.

4/13/2015 Monday
Woke around 6:45am. Ache in right side of head again today. Feel okay, sugar 95.
7:30am b/p 116/72 pulse 74
8am breakfast and pills Diovan and Toprol ½
Had coconut water and G2,
8:45am b/p 132/79 pulse 80 feel better, I guess because b/p is up.
Not good mentally this morning. Vascular Dementia? Or PMR/GCA?
10:45am. Prednisone 6 and ½ ninth day
Out around 12:30 for lunch, burger king at 1pm, then on to food shopping.
Home around 3pm., sugar 110. Felt bad the whole time out, dizzy off balance. Not good mentally, brain fog?
Eyes still swollen at 6:45pm
6 -6:30pm. sausage, broccoli, pasta, mushrooms olive oil, garlic, onion. Pills, verapamil, Plavix, aspirin.
Still not good mentally, hiccupping and burping a lot.
Right side of head ached today. GCA?
9pm bed to read, 9:30 protonix. Stayed awake till 10:45pm reading.

4/14/2015 Tuesday

Woke around 5:30am crazy dreaming then sweats, and feeling out of it. Sugar 78.

8am b/p 109/71 pulse 69

8:30 breakfast cereal ½ banana

b/p 115/76 pulse 70

9am b/p 120/78 pulse 69 took pills Diovan and Toprol ½

Have a brain this morning, and not as bad as yesterday's brain fog.

11am. Prednisone 6 and ½ tenth day

Out from 12 - 3pm, lunch, then store, haircut. Feeling pretty good, slightly agitated, nervous, but I'm out walking so the energy is going in that direction.

3pm home, back aches, feet and legs feel heavy, swollen.

4pm fell asleep on couch while reading.

6pm - 6:30 dinner, same as yesterday, sausage, pasta, broccoli, olive oil, garlic and pills, verapamil, Plavix, aspirin.

Feeling okay, hissing in right ear started after nap, 7:30pm Hissing is louder.

Bed around 9pm, protonix 9:30pm, sleep by 11pm

4/15/2015 Wednesday

Woke around 7am, good sleep last night. Woke maybe three times.

8am 137/68 pulse 72

Breakfast oatmeal

8:30 pills, Diovan and Toprol ½

Body aching a little this morning.

11am prednisone 6mgs first day drop ½ mg.

12:30pm. Skipped beats and lightheaded while standing cooking.

b/p 128/72 pulse 68 not good.

1:20pm eating lunch, pasta with tomato sauce, chicken, meatballs, and two cookies and milk.

Still not feeling good. Feeling scared, like other days. Not tired, but just not right.

3pm laid on couch to read and fell asleep, crazy dreams as at night.

Not good after nap, brain fog.

6 to 6:30pm dinner, same as lunch pasta, chicken, meatballs with sauce.

7:15pm still not good mentally. (I hate this feeling)

9pm bed to read 9:45pm protonix, 11pm sleep.

4/16/2015 Thursday

Woke around 6:30am. Slept well most of night, up twice. Out of bed around 7am

7:30am b/p 138/78 pulse 69

8am breakfast oatmeal and Diovan and Toprol ½

Throat again feels swollen and achy as the past few days.

11am Prednisone 6mgs second day down

Not bad today. Wheezing all day.

Around 1pm used inhaler, wheezing bad, and out of breath. In store I noticed I could breathe better, not out of breath. Home around 3pm.

On and off mentally not good today.

5:30 to 6:30pm Chills in right side of back while eating dinner. Took pills, verapamil, Plavix, aspirin.

Swollen throat also.

Tired tonight. Slept well, bed 9pm, protonix, 9:30pm sleep by 10:30pm.

4/17/2015 Friday

Woke at 2am, 4pm and 6. Stayed awake. Blood sugar 79, a little sweaty, but not bad.

8am b/p 122/78 pulse 69

Breakfast oatmeal, then pills, Diovan and Toprol ½.

Feeling nervous this morning, panic attack, afraid to be alone. Like years ago.

11:15am Prednisone 6mgs third day

12:30pm burger king, burger and fries, and dr. pepper.

2pm. Have company. A little nervous, b/p feels up, and face feels hot. Thinking okay, a little slow. Helping company do intricate work on computer.

5:30 – 6pm egg, waffle, ½ banana, cookie and milk, dinner, and pills, verapamil, Plavix, aspirin.

To bed early tonight, been up since 6am.

8:30pm. bed to read, 9:30pm protonix, 10:30am sleep.

4/18/2015 Saturday

6:30am Woke early, cold then sweats, not good mentally, grinding teeth, sugar 76. Had coconut water, better within half hour.

8am 119/78 pulse 70 still grinding teeth.

Breakfast cheerios and granola then b/p pills Diovan and Toprol ½

11am Prednisone 6mgs fourth day

An okay day so far.

3 – 5pm. fell asleep on couch while reading. Dreaming I saw words in front of my eyes, as I've seen before. The word travel real fast, as reading.

When I woke I was very cold with chills that I get up the right side of my back. Brain not right, confusion slight, just not right. Sugar 100. b/p 133/76 pulse 69. Temp. 97.7. pulse meter reads 68, 69, and oxygen at 95,96,97. Could it be oxygen that causes brain fog? Or problem with thinking? Or the low temperature? Or sugar?

6 to 6:30pm peanut butter and banana sandwich along with milk and cookie. Felt hour after eating.

Blood work from yesterday, SED rate 41, and CPR 9.1.

SED rate down which surprises me because I was in pain when I had test. Down from 47 in March.

8:15pm tired going to bed to read. 9:30 protonix. Sleep by 11pm.

4/19/2015 Sunday

Slept well last night, no sweats woke once around 4am.

6:30am awake, no sweats, feel okay.

7:30am sugar 80

b/p 113/79 pulse 74

8am breakfast b/p after 120/80 pulse 79 took pills, Diovan and Toprol ½

Feel okay this morning around 8:40am.

Wheezing since getting up, but no head problems.

10:45am. Prednisone 6mgs fifth day.

Okay this morning, and rest of early afternoon.

4 - 5pm fell asleep on couch while reading then woke with a start, slight headache over right eye, after dreaming. Confusion to time and place, Still in dream. b/p 120/80 pulse 72, pulse and oxygen meter 76 pulse oxygen 95,96,97. Sugar 108, temp 97.8.

5:45 - 6:15pm peanut butter and banana sandwich with milk and half Ensure, and pills, verapamil, Plavix, aspirin. Still feel out of it, brain wise from dream and still slight headache. Hopefully it will leave before bedtime.

Nervous, scared, teeth grinding. 9pm bed, 9:45 protonix, 11pm sleep, then woke around 12 midnight. Fell back to sleep then woke at 2 something, then again around 6am.

4/20/2015 Monday

Once up out of bed, wheezing right away. This seems to be happening every day.

6:30 - 7am b/p/ 126/84 pulse 72

Breakfast cereal cheerios and half banana.

8am pills Diovan and Toprol ½

Not bad this morning, feeling okay. Eyes lids swollen.

Out around 10am to store, walking good, not hurting or out of breath, even though I started wheezing earlier. Taking prednisone while in store with Ensure.

11:30am Prednisone 6mgs sixth day

12:30pm lunch, still feeling okay.

1:30pm. I notice I'm starting to feel not good, not quite brain confusion, but something is happening. Hissing in right ear starting, aching in right hip, left foot, leg swelling.

5:45 - 6:15pm dinner, egg, waffle with butter, grapes, cookies and milk. Pills, verapamil, Plavix, aspirin.

Feeling okay most of day 7:12pm now.

Brain wise, one slight problem today, not really brain fog or confusion.

Tired now, guess because I've been awake since 6am.

Bed by 9pm then protonix at 9:30, sleep around 10:30pm.

12 midnight, Woke cramping in foot and severe chills, couldn't get warm, put sweat shirt on trying to fall asleep. Feel asleep and woke with sweats, took sugar 75, drank some coconut water and lay awake. Eventually fell asleep, woke again with sweats 2am sugar 77. Stayed awake most of the night, sweats off and on. Fell asleep around 4am till 6am.

Bad night.

4/21/2015 Tuesday

Up around 7:30am, very tired from last night up all night, Sugar 80.

8am b/p 129/79 pulse 72

Breakfast cheerios, ½ banana, and grapes then pills Diovan and Toprol ½

11:20am Prednisone 6mgs seventh day

Feeling very cold this morning.

An okay day even though tired. Laid down around on couch and read but didn't fall asleep, even though tired.

Body aching more today, because of little sleep last night, I guess.

6 – 6:30pm peanut butter sandwich and ½ banana with milk and cookie. Pills verapamil, Plavix, aspirin.

Eyes swollen all day. Hope for sleep early.

9pm bed, 9:45pm protonix, lights out 10pm. Can't sleep, ¼ valium at 11pm, then fell asleep, woke at 3am, back to sleep till 6:30am

4/22/2015 Wednesday

Woke okay, sweats off and on, took sugar 83.

7:45 b/p 122/79 pulse 72

8am breakfast oatmeal then Diovan and Toprol ½.

10am Rheumy doctor.

He said stay on 6mgs of Prednisone for another two weeks, then go to five mgs. Have blood work again next month. I told him I was having trouble swallowing and throat felt soar. He told me to see my GP.

11am prednisone 6mgs eighth day.

To store after doctor, then home. aching body today.

6 – 6:30pm dinner, egg, waffle, grapes, one cookie and Ensure.

Feel tired even though napped around 3pm.

Hissing in right ear tonight.

8:45pm to bed to read. Protonix 10pm, sleep 10:30 ¼ valium.

4/23/2015 Thursday

Slept well last night, up 2 or 3 times but fell back to sleep.

Wake at 7am. Sugar 80.

b/p 117/75 pulse 72

8am breakfast

b/p 120/78 pulse 74 then pills Diovan and Toprol ½

9am feel okay this morning head wise so far.

11am Prednisone 6mgs eighth day

Worked typing all day until now at 3:30pm Brain worked well today. Did a lot of typing and thinking.

9pm bed, protonix 9:45pm, sleep 10:30pm. Woke around 12midnight, took ¼ valium fell back to sleep, woke at 4am, and stayed awake for a while.

Up at 6:30am.

***

Again I'll say, I know how boring this is reading, but if you have these diseases you're probably going through the same thing. Maybe you can write your story. Especially if you're living in the U.S.A. where little is known of this illness.

4/24/2015 Friday
7:30am 135/78 pulse 72
Wheezing as soon as out of bed.
7:30am Breakfast cereal then pills Diovan and Toprol ½
Out early 8am. Feeling heady, lightheaded, hissing in right ear and hearing is very acute in right ear, almost hurting when man with lawn mower came by, too loud for me.
11:30am Prednisone 6mgs ninth day with burger and fries and dr. pepper. Burger king.
Home around 12noon.
3pm still now hissing in right ear, eyes feel tired and swollen, belly still swollen from this morning along with feet. Ankles red.
5:30 to 6pm dinner, chicken salad, pills verapamil, Plavix, aspirin.
Very tired today, and slightly lightheaded.
Hissing in right ear all day along with chirping sound.
Wheezing all day.
8pm to bed to read then sleep. 9pm protonix then sleep.
Woke around 10pm, disoriented slightly. Sugar 88, back to sleep. Woke around 11:30pm. fast heart beat 105pulse, high b/p 150/90. Took ¼ valium then

laid awake reading until 1am, then slept. Woke around 4am, then 6:30am

4/25/2015 Saturday
Not a good night last night.
8am this morning, b/p 119/81 pulse 72
Breakfast cereal then pills Diovan and Toprol ½
11:20am Prednisone 5 ½ down first day.
Made smoothie, black cherries, blueberries, ½ banana, green romaine leaves, and carrot with coconut water.
Lunch rest of chicken salad from yesterday, cookies and milk.
3pm slight headache. Hearing very acute, right ear hissing lightly.
8pm still dizzy or light headed, nasal drip, and sneezing a lot. Don't like dizziness.
b/p 157/81 pulse 76, high.
Going to bed to read and rest. Slept well all night.
Woke two times.

4/26/2015 Sunday
Woke around 6am then fell back to sleep till 8am. Slept well all night, woke two times.
8:15am b/p 137/82 pulse 72
Breakfast oatmeal then pills Diovan and Toprol ½
Feeling well rested this morning, but still tired. No valium last night.

11am feeling slightly dizzy, lightheaded, like last night. Also nasal drip. Breathing is great, deep breaths, no wheezing all morning. Oxygen reading 97,98,99. b/p 124/78 pulse 69

11:10am Prednisone 5 ½ second day down. Had Ensure and two slices of ham.

Brain good this morning, thinking, so I'm writing, my favorite thing to do.

1pm lunch, steak and potato ½ cookie and milk.

Not good later in after noon, fell asleep around 4pm. while reading, even dreaming.

Woke not good, but not dizzy, as I earlier.

6:15 - 6:45pm. dinner, sausage, penna, broccoli, olive oil and garlic. With pills verapamil, Plavix, aspirin.

Tired tonight. Slept well, woke two times.

4/27/2015 Monday

Woke early around 6am after deep dream. Started sweating and not right brain wise. Checked sugar 77. Drank coconut water and hard piece of candy. Still not right and sweating a lot. Took b/p 156/90 pulse 79, then had to move bowels right away. This is happening a lot a notice, the feeling to move bowels upon waking. After I moved bowels I checked b/p 133/87 pulse 82. Checked pulse meter pulse high 70's and oxygen 95, 96, 97.

7:45am ate breakfast oatmeal then checked b/p 128/80 pulse 79 took pills Diovan and Toprol ½

10am. Going out, still not feeling well, head wise.

11am Prednisone 6mgs first day back to 6, off two days at 5 ½.

12pm back home. Lunch.

Felt better after lunch, still hissing in right ear, but better head wise.

3:20pm b/p 137/77 pulse 71 hissing in right ear.

6 - 6:30 dinner and pills.

Bed 9pm protonix, 9:45pm sleep by 10:30. Slept well all night, awake a few times but back to sleep. Bathroom one time.

4/28/2015 Tuesday

Woke around 7am slept well all night, no sweats.

8am b/p 116/75 pulse 70

Breakfast cheerios then pills Diovan and Toprol ½

Feeling okay, almost normal, whatever that is.

11:20am Prednisone 6mgs second up to six.

Feel good this morning, writing, have a brain. No Fog.

1:30pm lunch, made homemade chicken soup, feel good standing, nothing hurts as usual, back, legs, etc. had ice cream after lunch.

Around 3pm feeling slight confusion, not bad, but then got very sleepy, as drugged feeling. Laid on couch and fell asleep for ½ an hour.

Felt better when I woke. Still no pain in body.

6 - 6:30pm dinner, chicken salad with grapes, raisins, celery, on top of salad slice tomato. Also saltine crackers. Had ½ can dr. pepper.

7:30pm feel okay, slight hissing in right ear.

9pm bed to read, feel okay. 10:30pm protonix then sleep.

4/29/2015 Wednesday

Woke around 7am for the third time after a mixed up dream. Sweating a lot.

7:30am out of bed, bathroom, feel very shaky, legs, arms, whole body feels shaky. Also feel slight nausea. Very red lips, usually purple/red, looks like I have lipstick on.

Sugar 74.

Coconut water and sucked piece of candy.

8am sugar 104, feel better.

b/p 120/76 pulse 70

breakfast cheerios and ½ banana. Then took pills Diovan and Toprol ½

9:30am. feel okay but not great. Earlier episode takes the life out of me. Also notice upper leg muscles hurt.

11am As morning went on I felt really bad, head wise, front of head, including forehead heavy, also nasal drip, slightly light headed. Sugar 88. b/p 128/78 pulse 67. Oxygen 99, 98. Pulse low 61, 62.

11:20 Prednisone 6mgs. Taken with decaf coffee, slice bread with peanut butter, ½ banana.

12noon, still feeling not good, head wise, and nasal drip still there.

1:30pm lunch pasta, broccoli, sausage, garlic and olive oil. Ice cream.

Not good this afternoon either, heady, throat feels gritty. Possible from reflux last night. Belly very blown up today, especially later afternoon.

5:30 - 6pm dinner, soup and Ensure. Pills, verapamil, Plavix, aspirin. Bad belly. Doesn't hurt, just terribly blown up.

7:30pm still not good.

9pm bed to read, belly not good, blown up and indigestion. 9:30pm protonix. Sleep by 11.

Awake at 12midnight, awake again at 2, then at 5am.

4/30/2015 Thursday

Didn't sleep well last night.

Woke around 5am. sweats, hissing in ear, and mentally off. Sugar 75. Sucked piece of candy and coconut water. Stayed awake for forty-five minutes, then fell back to sleep. Crazy dreams after.

7:30am up. 8am b/p 128/84 pulse 69

Feeling okay.

8:30am breakfast cheerios and pills Diovan and Toprol ½

11:30am Prednisone 6mgs taken with ½ banana and slice bread with peanut butter, and milk.

Not great this morning, feel very cold, hissing in right ear, and slightly scared.

1pm 136/79 pulse 70. Sugar 108.

1pm to 5pm out. Feeling not bad, hissing still in right ear also feel closing of ear, muffled sounds.

Eye lids swollen all day.

5:30 to 6pm dinner, egg, waffle, pear, milk and cream cheese pie. Pills, Verapamil, Plavix, aspirin.

7pm Loud hissing in right ear.

7:30pm. surge of dizziness. B/p 153/84 pulse 69 Still hissing in ear.

Still dizzy when going to bed at 8:30pm feels like Vertigo.

½ valium

10pm protonix, awake a long time, then slept. Woke around 3am bad dreams, then sweats, Sugar 71. Sucked candy, coconut water, then fell asleep.

5/1/2015 Friday

Woke from dream 7:15am, when up to bathroom started sweating, shaky, took sugar 81.

8am b/p 124/84 pulse 70

Breakfast cheerios, ½ banana, 5 grapes.

8:30am pills Diovan and Toprol ½

Feeling not great, but not dizzy like last night.

10am physical therapy, tread mill twice, then leg and ankle exercise, pushing flat plate with weight on and leaning back was hard, especially in the belly area, legs and ankles, especially right leg, hip also weak and shaky.

11am prednisone 6mgs

After out food shopping. Home at 12 noon.

Okay most of day, not dizzy as last night.

5:30 - 6pm dinner and pills verapamil, Plavix, aspirin.

Feeling tired tonight and right foot hurts from exercises.

Hope for bed early tonight.

Went to bed and sleep at 9 after taking stomach pill Protonix.

Slept well, up one time 3am. Checked Sugar 81, then fell back to sleep.

5/2/2015 Saturday

Woke at 6am, and stayed awake. Feel good, not sweating or shaky.

7:30am b/p 116/74 pulse 62

8am breakfast cheerios, ½ banana and grapes.

8:30 b/p/ 122/80 pulse 71 Pills Diovan and Toprol ½

While eating breakfast I felt (not here) don't exist. Don't like this feeling.

Around 10am very sleepy, falling asleep in the chair. Laid down and feel asleep in bed for 45 minutes, dreaming.

11:30am Prednisone 6mg b/p 117/80 pulse 61

Not good today. Brain off, feeling not here, disoriented, confusion. Nasal drip, used spray Flonase. Head wise bad all day, except when I slept, morning and afternoon.

4-5pm slept on couch, sleepy as this morning.

6-6:30pm dinner, oatmeal ½ banana and raisins, Ensure and milk. Pills verapamil, Plavix, aspirin.

9pm bed, protonix 10:30, sleep. Slept well

5/3/2015 Sunday

Slept well, woke once or twice. No sweats, delirium or confusion.

7:15am woke. As soon as up walking wheezing started.

8am 119/81 pulse 74

Breakfast egg, waffle, ½ banana, coconut water and pills: Diovan and Toprol ½

9:20am feeling okay this morning, not out of it like yesterday.

Had swooshing sound in right ear, haven't had this in a while.

11am b/p 122/82 pulse 69

Working this morning, writing. Feel okay.

11:15am Prednisone 6mgs

1:30pm. lunch, feeling slightly depressed, or dislocated. Hate these feelings.

3:30pm reading on the couch, fell asleep, dreaming.

6-6:30pm dinner oatmeal then pills verapamil, Plavix, aspirin.

7:45pm Still feel sleepy. Left leg swollen all day.

9pm bed, 10pm protonix, then sleep.

Slept well all night, drank very little due to not waking up.

5/4/2015 Monday

Woke around 6:30am, bathroom, feel okay. Not sweating a lot.

7am sugar 91.

7:30am b/p 107/75 pulse 71 coconut water

Breakfast cheerios and ½ banana

8am b/p 135/78 pulse 77

Pills Diovan and Toprol ½

Not long after diarrhea cramps and then bathroom loose stool. Also dizzy.

Slight right forehead headache.

Not great this morning, intestinal problem, cold hands and body.

11:20am Prednisone 6mgs

12:30pm Burger King, the usual, burger fries and dr. pepper, then on to food shop.

Not great, head wise, as this morning. Swirling head.

2:30pm back home, having ice cream.

3:30pm feeling slightly better, except for belly blown up. Been since this morning's diarrhea.

Brain seems to feel better when b/p is higher and sugar is up. Maybe we need salt and sugar.

7:30pm b/p 140/86 pulse 68

Bed around 9pm, protonix 9:30pm. slept from 10:30pm to 2am. Then stayed awake all night, took ½ valium, and still stayed awake.

5/5/2015 Tuesday

7am out of bed, b/p 125/81 pulse 72

Breakfast cheerios and ½ banana.

8am Diovan and Toprol ½

GP this morning, 9:15, told me to see Rheumy and Endocrinologist for sugar testing.

I'm so tired of seeing different doctors for different things. What happen to one doctor treats all?

10:30am physical therapy, hurting and tired.

11:30am Prednisone 6mg with Ensure.

1pm lunch chicken and veggies cookie and ice cream.

2:30pm laying down to read, tired and hurting, right hip and lower back.

Fell asleep, dreaming, woke out of it, Sugar 108. Slight forehead headache, and running nose, clear liquid.

6 - 6:30pm dinner, peanut butter sandwich with ½ banana, cookie and milk. Pills, verapamil, Plavix, aspirin.

Achy from exercising today.

8:30pm to bed reading, 9:30pm protonix, then sleep around 10.

Slept well all night long, except for waking ice cold. Fell back to sleep. Woke maybe 3 times.

5/6/2015 Wednesday

Up at 7am, sweating a little. Woke to a bad dream.

8am breakfast 8:30 pills Diovan and Toprol ½

Feeling down, yet edgy.

11:15am Prednisone 5mg one down.

Better around lunch time but not great. Still nervous, cold and peeing a lot.

2:15pm lunch steak and veggies, ice cream and two pieces of chocolate.

4:15pm still nervous, peeing, hands cold. Sugar 106.

Bad day, very agitated, nervous, out of it mentally, almost delirium.

b/p slightly high later in day, 140/85 pulse 72

Felt better when eating dinner, chicken, pear, corn bread, Ensure. Pills verapamil, Plavix, aspirin.

7:30 indigestion, burning in middle of breast, regurgitation into throat.

Hissing in ear all day.

9pm bed, 9:30 protonix, then sleep at 10. Slept well, woke one or two times.

5/7/2015 Thursday

6:30am Woke throat feels cruddy, possibly because of last nights, stomach acid build up.

Out of bed 7am, shower first in over a month. Don't feel dizzy or lightheaded this morning.

8:15am b/p 125/78 pulse 72

Breakfast cheerios and ½ banana, and grapes.

8:45 Diovan and Toprol ½

Nasal drip, spray nose with saline solution, throat still cruddy.

Feeling okay mentally 10:15am., so far so good.

11am feeling slight headache over eye brows. Also mentally not great.

11:30am Prednisone 5mgs second day down. Had pill with one piece of bacon, ½ banana, and ½ ensure.

12:30pm out of Rheumy doctor's office. On to Wendy's for burger, fries, and dr. pepper. Why? Because I usually feel better after eating their burger, fries and dr. pepper.

Home around 2:30pm.

4:30pm headache coming back along with hissing in right ear.

Sugar 108, before eating.

6 to 6:30pm dinner, chicken salad, spinach, two oatmeal raisin cookies and milk. Pills Verapamil, Plavix, aspirin.

Headache not any better. Most of the day headache.

Tired tonight, right hip and groin hurts since physical therapy on Tuesday.

Hope to go to bed early.

7:30pm still have forehead headache and dizzy. Possibly vertigo, not sure. b/p 154/89 pulse 72 (high) had salt today.

Headache seems to come and go. Is this GCA coming back, even on prednisone?

8:30pm going to lay down and read.

9:30pm Valium ¼ then protonix twenty minutes later.

10:30pm sleep. Woke a number of times, don't know how many.

5/8/2015 Friday

Not a good night's sleep, woke many times, yet bathroom only one time around 3am.

6:30am woke and stayed awake.

7:30 b/p 125/81 pulse 75 Breakfast then b/p pills Diovan and Toprol ½

Feeling okay this morning other then headache upon waking. Forehead and top front of head.

10 – 11 physical therapy, did well.

11am prednisone 5mgs

3:30 to 4:30 fell asleep on couch woke having hissing in ear, and nasal drip.

6-6:30pm dinner and pills, verapamil, Plavix, aspirin.

7:30pm to bed.

9:15 protonix. Turn light off 9:30pm slept off and on.

5/9/2015 Saturday

7:15pm up out of bed. Feel okay.

8am b/p 119/76 pulse 71 Sugar 101

Breakfast and pills Diovan and Toprol ½

Sneezing this morning, and hissing in both ears.

11am prednisone 5mgs fourth day

Feeling okay this morning, except for nasal drip, have not used the saline spray, yesterday and today, no headache as of yet.11:30am

12:30 – 2pm went food shopping. Felt okay. Came home and cooked until 3:30. Back tired but other than that feel okay.

3:30 ate late lunch.

4:30 tired, lay on couch to read, feeling very cold, fell asleep for a half hour in an out of sleep. 6pm woke not good, very, very cold inside body chills, like I get at night in bed.

6:30pm bowl of oatmeal and raisins, glass of milk with pills, verapamil, Plavix, aspirin. Ears hissing, still cold. Eyes feel swollen.

8:30pm bed, very nervous again tonight, as last night. ¼ valium around 9pm. protonix 9:45pm, then sleep.

Slept then woke sweating. Cold prior to this.

5/10/2015 Sunday

7am out of bed. Sweating a lot this morning, took sugar 105. I notice at times I see things, bugs, crawling out of corner of my eyes. I've been seeing this a while, don't know if it's caused by prednisone?

8am b/p 114/67 pulse 71

Breakfast cheerios then pills Diovan and Toprol ½

Feeling not great this morning.

11am Prednisone 5mg fifth day

Turned out to be not a bad day, except for later afternoon. I got dizzy around 5:30pm.

6pm cheerios and Ensure for dinner with pills verapamil, Plavix, aspirin.

8:15pm Bed. Took ¼ valium 10pm, then again at 1:15am, can't sleep, keep waking up. Fell asleep, had crazy dreams, very vivid, but then forget them when awake.

5/11/2015 Monday

7am awake to stay. Lots of waking and sleeping last night, as usual, even with valium.

8am sugar 102, b/p 134/78 pulse 84

Breakfast oatmeal, had coconut water.

Pills Diovan and Toprol ½

Physical therapy today at 10am.

11am Prednisone 5mg sixth day

An okay day, even with company at the house.

8:30pm bed, 8:45 protonix then sleep.

Woke around 10pm totally out of it mentally, slept maybe an hour. Then awake and sleep most of night.

5/12/2015 Tuesday

6:30am awake yet tired from hardly any sleep last night.

Out of bed 7:15am, sugar 101. Feel tired, and hurting from exercise yesterday.

8am b/p 115/ 76 pulse 75

Breakfast oatmeal, grapes and ½ banana then pills diovan and Toprol ½

11:20 prednisone 5mgs seventh day

1:20pm lunch, pasta, sausage, broccoli, olive oil, garlic.

Bloated after eating and before, I guess due to oatmeal for breakfast.

2pm Feeling tired today due to little sleep last night and waking at 10pm out of it mentally.

Laid down awhile this afternoon and read, didn't fall asleep even though very tired.

6-6:30 dinner and pills, verapamil, Plavix, aspirin.

8pm indigestion, took ½ Tums, then laid in bed.

Feeling scared for some reason, mentally not good.

9:30pm protonix, then to sleep.

Crazy dreams most of night and into morning.

5/13/2015 Wednesday

4:30am woke ready to get up, but didn't. I stayed in bed on and off sleep, dreaming about spiders, then a moth which flew into my neck. I woke slapping the front of my neck at 7:45am. What causes these crazy dreams?

Out of bed right away. Sugar 100.

8am b/p 102/77 pulse 74

At first I felt okay but as I stayed upright I felt not good head wise.

Breakfast grapes, cherries, slice bread and butter, ½ piece of bacon and coffee (decaf) still b/p low

9am b/p 121/69 pulse 81 took pills Diovan/Toprol ½

Not good head wise, lightheaded. Drinking water and some G2.

12noon prednisone 5mgs eight day

An okay day, some mental confusion but not bad. Watched half a movie, then had company.

6-6:30pm dinner and pills verapamil, Plavix, aspirin.

Coughed a lot today. I had two nuts so I may get a migraine. Not so far at 7:30pm

Lower right side of spine hurt today to where I had to lie down. Also right lung hurt when breathing in.

8:30pm bed right lung hurts breathing in.

9:30 protonix, then sleep around 10:15pm

Woke off and on as always, dreamed about bugs again.

5/14/2014 Thursday
Woke around 7am to stay. A lot of waking and back to sleep last night, as usual.
Sugar 100.
8am b/p 114/78 pulse 73
Breakfast oatmeal, grapes, ½ banana
8:30 b/p 119/80 pulse 78
Pills diovan and Toprol ½
11:30am sugar 99 two hours after eating breakfast.
11:15am prednisone 5mgs ninth day
At this time had small slice of bread with butter, egg, small pastry.
12noon out to store and haircut, feeling slightly lightheaded.
3pm back home, sugar 115.
Had dinner early sausage, pasta, ice cream
An okay day.
6-6:30pm avocado, chicken, ½ banana and pills, verapamil, Plavix, aspirin.
Hissing in right ear, first today.
8:30pm bed to read, 9:30 protonix, then sleep around 10:30pm
Slept well through the night, awake one time.

5/15/2015 Friday

Woke at 5am with cramp in right foot and ankle, then cramp under left breast when trying to get up. Didn't feel good. Went to bathroom and took sugar 90. Drank some coconut water. Kept feeling bad, then worse. Brain felt off. B/p felt high on wrist cuff. 140's Stayed awake.

7:15am b/p 191/90 pulse 90 ate breakfast to take b/p pills Diovan and Toprol ½

Back to bed to rest. Then I started to shake (tremor) in right leg then right arm, mostly right side. Brain still didn't feel right.

By 9am I was bad. Went to ER Hospital.

Very high B/P and bad shakes. Shakes lasted long, maybe two hours, settling down slowly.

They didn't do blood work until two hours later. Nurse was terrible. She couldn't draw blood or put a needle in to give me fluids. After four tries I ask her to get someone else. Waiting more time for someone to come. Then she asked for urine much later.

They sent me for a CTScan of the brain, (negative) EKG (okay) Chest x-ray (okay).

B/P went down to 140's finally, but then back up to 170's.

I left. b/p 170's they told me to take the other half of my Toprol at home.

2:30pm. Toprol ½ home.

Had something to eat for lunch

3:30pm took Prednisone 5mgs tenth day (very late)

6pm b/p 120/58 pulse 71

6:30 ate sandwich peanut butter and ½ banana with milk and cookie.
Will take verapamil later before bed.
9pm bed to read.
10:30pm Verapamil, and Tums then sleep, NO Protonix first in a long time.
Didn't sleep, but rested.

5/16/2015 Saturday
8am 123/76 pulse 72 Breakfast then pills Diovan and Toprol ½ Feel okay.
Feeling okay today.
11am Prednisone 5mgs eleventh day
12:30 tired and slightly heady, pain on right upper side of head, for like an ache, even when pressed down.
135/76 pulse 68
3pm tried laying down, but can't fall asleep, yet tired.
Just saw blood work from yesterday's Emergency room visit.
SED rate 53, as high as when I started on Prednisone. Now What?
Could be the cause of yesterday's head feeling and today's pain in head.
5pm feeling like I did yesterday.
5:30pm b/p 170/85 pulse 72 not well, heady, and slightly dizzy. b/p just spiked up for no reason, no salt. I have felt my belly bloated as the day went on.

Started to feel tremors again also, slightly in right arm and hand.

5:45pm Milk with pills, Verapamil, Plavix, aspirin.

6pm ¼ valium

6:45pm b/p 140/75 pulse 69, feeling better.

7:30pm b/p 150/84 pulse 72 back up, hissing in ear and right side of headaches.

If this stays up I'll take an extra ½ of Toprol tonight.

Bad night awake most of the night. b/p ran high.

5/17/2015 Sunday

5:30am woke sweating, and heart beating fast. Took b/p 176/87 Pulse 99 took Diovan and Toprol whole pill instead of half I usually take with Ensure.

I notice when this happens I have to move bowels every time.

7am b/p 157/80 pulse 74

9am took potassium, calcium, magnesium vitamin, see if it helps b/p go down.

10am b/p 137/81 pulse 69

11:15am prednisone 6mgs went up one because of SED rate 53 high.

12noon b/p 150/80 pulse 68

Laying down resting mostly this morning.

2:30pm 124/77 pulse 68 first time b/p down, feel almost normal, relaxed.

Slept half an hour prior to this.

Lunch/dinner pasta and chicken, little ice cream.

Slight hissing in right ear.

6pm b/p 145/85 pulse 66

Oatmeal and pills, verapamil, Plavix, aspirin.

Feel better today, very tired from little sleep the last two nights. Wonder if it's due to the increase in prednisone? b/p still running high though.

7:30pm Hissing in ear loud tonight.

Hope to go to bed around 8pm

Belly blown up. Slept the whole night, woke once or twice, then back to sleep.

5/18/2015 Monday

Woke around 7am feeling okay, then half hour later didn't feel right. Head bothering me, not dizzy, but unsteady on my feet, off balance.

7:30am b/p 154/77 pulse 80 (high)

Breakfast and pills Diovan and Toprol (whole pill instead of half) Don't know what's making b/p high.

10:30am b/p 145/78 pulse 69

11am prednisone 6mgs second day back to six taken with Ensure.

General Practitioner, different doctor, same office. This GP seems annoyed at me, told me take my blood pressure meds same time every day. I disagreed. "Cardiologist told me to take it when my b/p is 120 or over."

GP gave me script for cortisol and SED rate. I went to Hospital for blood work. Waited an hour and more, then discussed I went to Burger King for burger, fries, and dr. pepper.

Then on to store for shopping. Feeling better.

3:30pm home b/p 127/81 pulse 74 (normal, finally)

Why do I feel better after going to burger king?
5:30pm b/p 133/79 pulse 64 (normal finally)
6-6:30 pills, verapamil, Plavix, aspirin
Hoping to go to bed early tonight.
Tums, indigestion, sleep by 10:30pm. Woke around 1am. hissing in ear.

5/19/2015 Tuesday
7:30am up, awake since 7am.
139/82 pulse 62
Breakfast cheerios, ½ banana, grapes, coconut water.
Eye sight bad, very blurred.
8:30am 120/75 pulse 69
b/p pills Diovan and Toprol ½ pill.
11am b/p 137/81 pulse 64.
11:15am Prednisone 6mgs third day.
Not bad this day, but not great.
1:30pm b/p 126/77 pulse 70
Lunch, steak, potato, ice cream.
Headache on top of head, first in a while, nasal drip and throat problem.
3:15pm still not great head wise.
5:30pm b/p 128/81 pulse 74
6-6:30pm dinner and pills, verapamil, Plavix, aspirin.
Dizzy surge while eating dinner. Headache again on top of head, into forehead above eyebrows. Also nasal drip, and throat crud. Also seeing white light moving on side of left eye.

Haven't had anything to give me an ocular migraine, no nuts.
Bad night (all) night.
High blood pressure. 8pm high b/p ½ Toprol

***

This is how it went for almost three years. Up and down on prednisone. I got down to 3mgs, then back up, until I got down to a ½ mgs. for a month. It was then I decided to go off prednisone. Doctors told me no, but I couldn't stand the drug anymore and felt it was causing more problems than what I started out with.

From online support groups for GCA/PMR, mostly women went through the same illness I did. Some lost sight in one eye because prednisone dose was not high enough. I guess I took my chances. I'm thankful I didn't lose my eye sight and it's back to where it was years ago. Some developed bleeding ulcers and other illnesses, related to Kidneys, Adrenal glands, and Heart.

I still see the eye doctor. Instead of every three months, I see him once a year. Black spots in front of eyes gone, pain behind right eye gone, eyesight better, not blurred or fuzzy. I also see the stomach doctor for colonoscopy and endoscopy every year, making sure rawness in my intestines, stomach and esophagus are gone.

I don't see the Rheumy anymore, Neurologist or Endocrinologist (Thyroid nodules are gone)

I see a General Practitioner who specializes in muscles and nerves. He's offered me 5mgs of prednisone for pain in hips, upper thighs and arms but I've refused. I'd rather have pain then be on prednisone.

I no longer have headaches on the right side of my head or jaw ach on the same side. I no longer feel I'm having a stroke.

I see the cardiologist who says, "you're doing fine." Especially after having a stress test.

Only drugs I take are blood pressure pills which have decreased to two plus Plavix, one in the morning and two at dinner for VTac. At night I take ½ valium for sleep and pain relief in neck, hips and arms.

Recently SED rate came back 58 and I decided against taking prednisone. The GP didn't push it. All he said, "you can take 5mgs just for pain."

My heart goes out to all those who have PMR or GCA and know what they are going through.

Recently I've been diagnosed with breast cancer so I guess this will be another adventure within the large Adventure of life.

***

This went on and on: reduce prednisone, then flare, increase prednisone.

Dizziness
Itching hands
Brain Fog, one doctor calls it.

Not here feeling.
Confusion
Disconnected
Sweating
Chills
Nausea
Diarrhea
Constipation
Blind spots in sight
Pain in head, forehead, jaw.
Pain in back of neck
Ache in upper thighs
Ache in upper arms
Spasms and Cramps in muscles
Burning stomach
Hissing in right ear
Lightheadedness
Crazy dreams
Seeing bugs crawling on the sides of my eyes
Shakes, jittery, all through body.
Sides of face didn't feel right. I had over 5 CTscans
of brain, checking for stroke.
SED rate up higher dose of prednisone taken and it
would go down.
Someone in England wrote me saying, "Why didn't
they put you on 60mgs of Pred. in the beginning?"
This leads me to believe the medical profession in
U.S. doesn't know much about PMR and GCA.

I've been on too many drugs: antidepressant,
anxiety, antibiotics, stomach acid, vertigo drugs that

make you sleep, neuropathy pills for feet pain, burning and numbness.

Again, I hope this helps others.

The End

Printed in Great
Britain
by Amazon